How to Choose a
MEDICAL
SPECIALTY

Fifth Edition

Anita D. Taylor, M.A.Ed.
Assistant Dean for Student Development
Associate Professor
Department of Family Medicine
Oregon Health & Science University
School of Medicine
Portland, Oregon

CONTRIBUTORS

The Couples Match

SCOTT THOMAS HADDEN, M.D.
TANIE HOTAN, M.D.
   Private Practice, Aumsville, Oregon

RIMA CHAMIE, M.D.
MATTHEW D. WAGNER, M.D.
   Portland, Oregon

Military Programs

DEVON GREER, M.D.
   Madigan Army Medical Center, Tacoma, Washington

BRITTANY MILLARD-HASTING, M.D.
   David Grant Medical Center, Travis Air Force Base, California

JESSE SCHONAU, M.D.
   Naval Hospital, Camp Pendleton, California

Mill City Press, Inc.
212 3rd Avenue North, Suite 290
Minneapolis, MN 55401
612.455.2294
www.millcitypublishing.com

ISBN-13: 978-1-938223-65-5
LCCN: 2012916481

Printed in the United States of America

Contents

Part 3: EMERGING SPECIALTY AREAS

Part 4: PRACTICE OPTIONS

Part 5: AFTER YOU HAVE CHOSEN A SPECIALTY

Preface

THIS YEAR IS THE 26TH ANNIVERSARY OF THE PUBLICATION OF the first edition of *How to Choose a Medical Specialty*. In 1986 I wrote this book because medical students were apprehensive about having to choose their lifetime careers without the facts they felt they needed to make an informed decision. Seven years later the second edition of this book was written as an adjunct to the increasing availability of resources developed by medical school administrators, such as career advisory systems and programs on choosing a medical specialty and applying for residency positions. In 1997 the Association of American Medical Colleges (AAMC) and the American Medical Association (AMA) announced a joint initiative to "develop strategies, materials and real-time data to assist students with the process of career planning," making extensive use of web-based technology. Clearly, the medical education system was paying attention to the important issue of medical student career choice, but the 3rd edition, published in 1999 with a revised printing in 2001, was needed to address the rapidly changing medical marketplace and expanding specialty and practice location options. After completing the 4th edition of the book in 2003, I decided that because students and faculty had access to information on the medical specialties and residency applications on multiple websites this would be the final edition. And yet, as I travel around the country speaking to medical students and faculty members on their campuses and at national medical student meetings, I find a continuing need for material from one authoritative source in hard copy that can serve as both an information source and a personal workbook. This is why there is now a 5ᵗʰ edition.

The goal of the book remains the same as in the first edition: to serve as a guide to self-discovery and a resource for information on the specialties in medicine based on physicians' comments and authoritative references.

The book continues to offer specific guidelines and individual worksheets for students to complete as they learn about the specialty options in medicine. Filling in these pages has helped students sort out their thoughts and feelings as they recorded their attitudes, values, and preferences. Therefore, in Part 1 of the book, I have retained the guidelines and worksheets for you, the reader, to complete. I believe that this activity will give you a sense of control over your decision making and the book will become an important part of your life narrative. Also, in Part 1, I have discussed the current controversy about workforce projections. At the end of this chapter are the data from the graduating classes of 2010 and 2011 concerning their specialty preference pre-first year and at graduation. This is in response to an increasing need to prepare students for specialty decisions and residency applications in light of increasing class sizes and an unchanging number of residency positions.

Part 2 of the book describes the 26 American Board of Medical Specialties (ABMS) approved medical specialties and selected subspecialties. I have added new information and references in each of the chapters from the fourth edition. Part II has an updated summary of focused data called, "Fast Facts," at the beginning of each specialty chapter, a feature requested by student readers.

Part 3 continues to focus on the emerging specialty areas of addiction medicine, administrative medicine, adolescent medicine, critical care medicine, geriatric medicine, hospice and palliative care medicine, sports medicine and women's health, updating information on each.

The addition of a new section of the book, Practice Options, Part 4, in the third edition, has proved to be right on target. Physicians either immediately after completing their training years or in mid-career are seeking practice settings that fit their non-medical as well as their medical interests. I believe that the type of practice setting you desire needs to be considered when choosing your specialty. I have updated information that discusses practice options both in clinical and non-clinical settings as well as "niche" and part-time opportunities. Included in this section are the opportunities for those with combination degrees, such as MD/JD, MD/MPH or MD/PhD.

Part 5 updates information on the process of applying to residency programs, including the Electronic Residency Application System (ERAS). There is new information in the chapter Military Programs and I have retained the popular chapters The Couples Match, What Happens If I Do Not Match?, and Changing Specialties During Residency and Afterwards.

As I discuss specialty choice with medical students, I am increasingly aware of the important role of the spouse or partner in this process. I urge you to openly include him or her in this very important step in your life, allowing a sharing of feelings and perceptions as you support each other in your endeavors.

I encourage readers to continue to write, telephone, or talk to me about suggestions for the book. I thank the more than 350 physicians who shared their perceptions on the various areas of medicine, the residency directors and faculty members at the Oregon Health Sciences University (OHSU) who reviewed the specialty chapters and gave their thoughts on residency application, and the numerous individuals in the medical associations and specialty societies who have suggested resources and shared information. I especially appreciate the assistance of Molly Osborne, Ph.D., M.D., OHSU Associate Dean for Student Affairs. At the Student Doctor Network I thank Laura Turner for her initial contact and proposal for me to write a 5th edition. And to Robert B. Taylor, M.D., my personal and professional partner, thank you for being there at all times.

Anita D. Taylor

How to Use This Book

THE BOOK IS DIVIDED INTO FIVE MAIN SECTIONS. PART 1 HAS material discussing the challenges facing you as you choose a specialty and offers practical guidelines and worksheets to aid in decision making.

Part 2 gives comprehensive information on the specialties and subspecialties for which there is board certification approved by the American Board of Medical Specialties (ABMS). Each chapter gives factual information about the specialty and draws a composite picture of its practitioners. The composite is based on a questionnaire completed by physicians from a variety of geographic locations, types of practice settings, and professional backgrounds. An effort has been made to have representation from both male and female physicians in each field more or less in proportion to the actual numbers in that specialty, and to have contributors who are board certified in their specialty. There is a wide spectrum of ages, ranging from 29 to 75. The questions asked were suggested by medical students as pertinent in helping them to compare themselves with the practitioners of various specialties. To help you get the full benefit from this book, let's review the format of the chapters in Part 2.

At the beginning of each of the "specialties" chapters "Fast Facts" gives statistical information on residency/fellowship training and practice data as well as what program directors value highly in an applicant. The information for this and other sections of the book is compiled from the following major sources:

National Resident Matching Program 2011 Match Data

Results of the 2010 NRMP Program Director Survey, May 2010

Charting Outcomes in the Match, 4th edition. Prepared by the National Resident Matching Program and the Association of American Medical Colleges, August 2011.

The 2011 Medical Education issue of the *Journal of the American Medical Association*

2010 American Board of Medical Specialties Guide to Medical Specialties

Physician Characteristics and Distribution in the US 2011 Edition, American Medical Association

Information on what residency directors look for in applicants is from two major sources: Results from the 2010 Program Directors Survey, a National Resident Matching Program (NRMP) research report and a national survey of residency directors. [1]

General Information. Each chapter begins with a general description of the specialty, which may include historical data, information about the scope of activity, and commonly held beliefs about the specialty.

Residency Information. This section gives information about residency program requirements and the numbers of positions available.

American Board of Medical Specialties Certification. Twenty-one primary and three conjoint examining and certifying boards issue certificates attesting to an individual's qualifications to practice a particular specialty. The primary objective of specialty boards is to assure the quality of medical education and care; the certificate issued is not to be confused with a medical degree, license, or legal document.

The first specialty board, for ophthalmology, was organized in 1916. The most recent, for medical genetics, was approved in 1993. Subspecialists in surgery have formed their own specialty boards, whereas medical subspecialists are awarded certificates by the American Board of Internal Medicine (ABIM). Each specialty has different requirements for residency training and admission to the examination for certification. These requirements are included here since this is now the norm for physicians and you should be aware of the requirements for ABMS certification to help you make informed long-range decisions. More and more, physicians are finding that in legal and financial terms the effort to achieve ABMS certification is worthwhile. If medical liability issues arise, a physician's position is strengthened by being certified. Also, managed care organizations have excluded physicians without ABMS credentials.[2]

Supply and Projections. Though you should not base your specialty choice decision solely on the basis of projections of physician supply, you should be familiar with this topic. The major sources of data for this section of the chapters are studies on the physician workforce in the United States. Some of the studies were undertaken by individual specialty societies and others were done by individual researchers and recruiting companies and offer data on more than one specialty. The major sources of information on the entire profession of medicine are the Council on Graduate Medical Education report in 2005, [3] and the research reported by Cooper et.al in 2002 and 2009. [4-5]

Past and present supply and activity statistics are from the individual specialty boards, the American Medical Association's publication Physician Characteristics and Distribution in the United States 2011 edition, [6] and referenced articles from the medical literature.

Economic Status and Types of Practice. Three income studies and data from a published article are the major source of data in this section of each chapter—the Medical Group Management Association (MGMA) Physician Compensation and Production Survey, 2011 report based on 2010 data; The Medscape Physician Compensation Report 2011; and the Merritt, Hawkins & Associates 2011 review of Physician Recruitment Incentives [7-10] Keep in mind that economic reimbursement systems in medicine change, and that the high-paying tertiary care specialties may not always be so financially rewarding because of increased competition, the cyclical emphasis on ambulatory care settings, and the federal government's restructuring of Medicare fees through the Resource Based Relative Value Scale (RBRVS).

Information on types of practice was drawn from answers to the questionnaires, as well as from representatives of specialty societies. Here also, change is predicted as many see more physicians choosing to work part-time and a variety of practice settings and styles.

Further Information. The name, address, telephone number, and internet address of the major specialty society are cited, as well as helpful resources for medical students pertinent to the specialty.

A Composite Picture. The composite of each specialty was drawn from the answers to the questionnaires. "Respondent" refers to a physician who gave that specific answer to the question. By not attributing comments to specific individuals, some degree of anonymity has been preserved; this was my agreement with the contributors. The questionnaire used as a basis for these chapters is printed in the Appendix.

Why Choose This Specialty? The composite picture under this heading derives from answers to numbers 1, 2, 11, and 12 of the questionnaire: when the choice was made, what was attractive about the specialty, what other specialties had you considered and why were they not chosen, and what specialty was and is not attractive? It would be helpful to compare yourself carefully to the responses to this last question. It is often easier to identify the specialties you do not like than to determine one favorite, and, in this question, both sides of the issue are addressed. Look for specific similarities of interests between you and the respondents in each specialty.

What Do You Like Most About This Specialty? The responses will give a clue as to what you will find enjoyable about the work of this specialty. Evaluate the satisfactions you need from your work activity in relation to those described by the respondents. Is patient contact important? Do you feel energized in the operating room? Do you look forward to—or dread—the responsibility of being in charge? Do you like to be presented with new challenges or would you prefer having a fairly well-defined set of answers to problems presented?

One source of career satisfaction data is from a 2002 article [11] reporting data from the Community Tracking Survey of 12,474 physicians (response rate 65 percent) from the late 1990s. There are two satisfaction variables: very satisfied and dissatisfied. The mean for all specialties combined was 42.3 percent for "very satisfied" and 17.6 percent for "dissatisfied." The statistically significant results on specialties are the following:

"Very Satisfied" High Percentages	"Dissatisfied" High Percentages
Geriatric internal medicine	Otolaryngology
Neonatal-perinatal medicine	Obstetrics-gynecology
Dermatology	Ophthalmology
Pediatrics	Orthopedic surgery
	Internal medicine

Even though more than 70 percent of US physicians reported being satisfied or very satisfied with their medical careers, nearly 1 in 5 are dissatisfied. The highest percentage of "very satisfied" are over age 65 and, to a lesser degree, young physicians. No differences were found between men and women. Specific information on specialties reported is presented in the individual specialty chapters.

What Do You Like Least About This Specialty? Here the responses will give you clues as to what your frustrations will be if you choose this specialty. Some complaints, such as "paperwork" and "bureaucracy," are common to almost every specialty, but they seem to be more bothersome to those physicians who value personal independence highly. Other aspects, such as "no continuity of care" or "office routine," must also be evaluated in terms of your own temperament. Respondents generally stated that they found negative aspects of their specialty to be minor inconveniences. To you, they may be major frustrations.

What Is Your Typical Daily Schedule? Some specialties have a less typical daily schedule than others. First, you should ask yourself if you like a typical daily schedule. How much of a schedule is tolerable? Or intolerable? The responses provide information about the time commitment made, the type of activities performed, and how much is expected professionally during evenings and weekends. Although it is true that you can work as much or as little as you like in any specialty (radiologists can go to the hospital and read x-rays all night if they really want to), some fields will require a less structured time commitment than others. The surgeon cannot be sure that an operation will be finished at a predetermined time; the emergency room physician knows when a shift will end. You need to have some reasonable expectations as to how much time you are willing to spend in the practice of medicine and match that with the typical daily schedule in each specialty.

What Abilities and Talents Are Important in This Specialty? No matter how motivated you are to work in a specific specialty area, you may not have the talents and abilities required for success in that field. In some cases you may be able to develop the talent or ability, such as learning good management and listening skills in preparation for a career in physical medicine and rehabilitation, but you may not be able to acquire manual dexterity or good eye-hand coordination needed to perform surgery, or the physical requirement of normal color vision which is a prerequisite for ophthalmology. Included in the responses are areas of training that are related to personal interests and skills, such as "a strong scientific orientation with interest in anatomy and histology" for pathology or "piloting aircraft" for aerospace medicine.

What Personality Traits Best Characterize This Specialty? This question is closely related to the previous one. The key word in assessing yourself in relationship to this question is *temperament.* Anyone can practice almost any specialty in medicine, aside from some physical limitations. In some specialties, however, you will feel more comfortable than in others, and it will be easier for you to do the required work. Your own individual personality (or temperament) will be the key factor. In addition to the responses of the physician contributors, I have drawn upon Mary H. McCaulley's "Application of the Myers-Briggs Type Indicator to Medicine and Other Health Professions" as a resource.[12]

What Advice Would You Give to Medical Students Interested in This Specialty? Because so many respondents said they would advise a student to "take a clerkship in the field," "talk to physicians in the specialty," or in similar ways get first-hand experience of the specialty considered, this advice can apply to all specialties. Each chapter includes advice *specific* to the specialty under consideration.

What Are the Future Challenges to This Specialty? In addition to published material about the future of each specialty in terms of personnel, income, and practice styles, it would be interesting for you to read what practicing physicians see as the future trends in their specialties. It is important to measure your expectations of a career field in relation to these responses.

Job Values of This Specialty. In a pretest, physicians listed their job values; their top choices are listed below. Each respondent was asked to choose *four* of the following job values that are most important to him or her:

_____ Creativity	_____ Decision making	_____ Working with my hands
_____ Good income	_____ Prestige	_____ Working with my mind
_____ Variety	_____ Achievement	_____ Taking care of people
_____ Security	_____ Working with people	_____ Feedback from others
_____ Independence	_____ Sufficient time off	

At this time, check off your top four choices from this list, or complete this quiz online at http://www.sdn.net. As you read through each chapter you will be able to compare your job values with those of the respondents in each specialty.

It is also important to know which job values were *not* chosen by *any* of the respondents because this may give you a clue as to what you should not expect from the specialty. For example, no one in aerospace medicine chose "good income," "working with my hands," "taking care of people," or "feedback from others" as a job value; in dermatology, no one chose "prestige."

Summary Profile of This Specialty. For each specialty ten tendencies are cited. These have been derived from the short-answer statements in number 14 of the questionnaire (see the Appendix) as well as from information on the questionnaires. You will be asked to compare yourself with the tendencies listed on a numerical scale to provide a score at the end of each specialty chapter. The higher your score, the more similar you are to the respondents in that specialty; the lower your score, the less similar you are. You may record your individual chapter scores in the Appendix. When you finish Part 2 some specialties should seem to offer opportunities satisfying to you—and these should be investigated further.

Part 3 discusses emerging areas of specialty interest. This section has been written in response to student requests for information about medical fields that are certified by more than one primary board (such as geriatrics and critical care) or that may be practiced with training in any of a variety of specialties (such as administrative medicine). The key question from students was, "How do I prepare myself to offer special expertise in these areas either in a full-time practice or as an adjunct to one of the traditional specialties?" Suggestions for other areas that might be included in future editions are welcome.

The discussion of these emerging areas of specialty interest follows a format similar to that used in Part 2, that is, it offers information about the specialties and the physicians who practice in these fields. Information about training pathways for their practice focus and advice for students interested in pursuing similar interests are included.

Part 4 focuses on practice options and outlines clinical and non-clinical pathways you can follow. The goal is to learn how to integrate your preferences of where and how you live and your interests outside medicine with your specialty choice. To this end I have responded to students' requests for information on international medicine, wilderness medicine, research opportunities, and hospitalists' careers, as well as adding a plethora of other pathways you can follow.

Part 5, After You Have Chosen a Specialty, is comprised of six chapters. There is information on the NRMP, the military programs, the couples match, shared residencies, and independent matching programs, as well as what happens if you do not match. A chapter discusses changing specialties during or after residency. Resources for these chapters include medical students, residents, and the annual Directory of Graduate Medical Education Programs published by the American Medical Association.

REFERENCES

1. Green M, Jones P, Thomas JX. Selection criteria for residency: results of a national program directors' survey. *Acad Med* 2009; 84(3):362-367.
2. Wallace AP. HMOs and physicians without board certification. Letter to the Editor. *N Engl J Med* 1993; 328(20):1501–1502.
3. Council on Graduate Medical Education. *Physician Workforce Policy Guidelines for the U.S. for 2000 – 2020.* Rockville, MD: U.S. Department of Health and Human Services; 2005.
4. Cooper RA, Getzen TE, McKee HJ, Laud P. Economic and demographic trends signal an impending physicians shortage. *Health Affairs* 2002; 21(1): 140-154.
5. Cooper RA, Getzen TE, Johns M.M.E. Physicians and Their Practice Under Health Care Reform, A Report to the President and the Congress prepared on behalf of The Physicians Foundation, September 9, 2009.
6. Physician Characteristics and Distribution in the US, American Medical Association, 2011.
7. Physician Compensation Report 2011 Medscape. Accessed June 16, 2011 at www.medscape.com
8. MGMA Physician Compensation and Production Survey: 2011 Report based on 2010 data. Englewood, CO.
9. 2011 Annual Review of Physician Recruitment Incentives, Merritt, Hawkins & Associates, Irving, TX, 20

10. Leigh JP, Tancredi D, Jerant A, Kravitz RL. Physician wages across specialties. *Arch Intern Med* 2010; 170 (19): 1728-1734.

11. Leigh JP, Kravitz RL, Schembri M, Samuels SJ, Mobley S. Physician career satisfaction across specialties. *Arch Intern Med* 2002; 162:1577-1584.

12. McCaulley MH. Application of the Myers-Briggs Type Indicator to Medicine and Other Health Professions, Monograph I. Gainesville, FL: Center for Applications of Psychological Type, 1978.

PART 1

THE CHALLENGE OF SPECIALTY CHOICE

Planning Your Specialty Choice

SOME OF YOU READING THIS BOOK HAVE ALWAYS WANTED TO be physicians. Others made the decision to go to medical school during college or later. Can you remember when and how you set your goal of becoming a physician? Perhaps a personal or family illness has had some influence. Or maybe your family's physician is the person you most admire and wish to emulate in your life. For some there may be one or more physicians in your family—your choice of medicine may be preordained by family expectations or freely chosen as an admirable vocation. Or medicine may seem to offer a life of prestige and wealth.

All of you have made short-term choices: for example, the college or graduate school you attended, the major area of study you chose, the medical schools to which you applied. Now, however, you are faced with what seems to be a long-term choice—what you will do during your career in medicine.

> *When I first arrived here at medical school I just wanted to be a doctor. I didn't know anything about specialties.*
> *—Junior medical student*

Students often have vague ideas about the process of becoming a physician. The Association of American Medical Colleges' Section for Student Programs annually administers the Matriculating Student Survey, a questionnaire which includes the query: "How important were the following factors in your choice of medicine as a career goal?" Most recently, the top two answers are "opportunity to make a difference" and "educate patients about health." Also at the top of the list are "continued contact with patients," "exercise of social responsibility," "critical thinking," and "intellectual challenge." You may be able to identify with one of these themes more than with the others, and it may be reflected in your specialty preference. Or, you may feel that all these aspects of medicine are equally important in your life.

A few students have made firm decisions concerning specialty choice prior to entering medical school; most vacillate and make a commitment sometime during their third year; some are unsure at the time of graduation and hope to decide during residency. Even children of physicians may not know much about the various career options—their physician parent(s) may know little about the specialties outside his or her area of interest.

In the past decade there has been an increased emphasis on career planning in many areas of business and the professions. Medical students have for many years realized that such planning is especially desirable in the process of choosing a medical specialty. Three specific factors have been instrumental in creating the need for medical specialty choice counseling: the increased number of options, time pressures, and the projected surplus of physicians in some specialties.

Increased Options. The Council on Medical Education of the American Medical Association (AMA) and the American Board of Medical Specialties (ABMS) have approved 21 primary and three conjoint examining and certifying boards. In addition, certification in subspecialty fields is conferred by individual boards or boards conjointly, such as in geriatrics by both the American Board of Family Medicine and the American Board of Internal Medicine. Although almost all of the 24 certifying boards were established prior to 1949, the number of residency positions offered has steadily increased, reflecting the trend toward specialization in medicine. Even the generalist became a specialist with the establishment of the American

Board of Family Practice in 1969. In 1945 there were 8930 residency positions available in all specialties. Twenty years later, in 1965, the number had increased to 38,979.[1] In 2010-2011, there were 111,586 residents in 8,967 ACGME-Accredited and Combined Specialty Graduate Medical Education programs. Of these, 25,292 were first year residents with no prior residency experience.[2]

Time Pressures. A medical school dean of student affairs has said that one of his greatest frustrations is trying to convince students to relax in their quest for a medical specialty. The earlier this question is faced, he thinks, the greater is their anxiety.

I disagree. By actively becoming involved in self-study, information gathering, and setting timelines, you can achieve a sense of control over the process. Finding a purpose in life involves establishing your occupational identity and is, therefore, related to choosing a specialty for the physician. While it is true that in some peoples' lives chance occurrences may lead them to a certain specialty that turns out to be just right, this is not often the case. Planning, as long as it is done with some degree of flexibility, seems to be the wisest course of action.

Medical students need to make some commitment to a specialty by the beginning of their fourth year—the time they apply for residency training. In addition, for some specialties, it is important to do a clerkship at your top choice program early in your fourth year. This is true especially in the competitive programs located in highly desirable geographic areas which attract large numbers of applicants, such as an orthopaedic surgery residency in the Southern California area. It may be necessary to apply for this clerkship during your second year of medical school, which may advance your timeline.

Early planning is recommended for the military match program and for other specialties with match programs (in 2011 these are child neurology, ophthalmology, and urology). These match programs are concluded by January or February, one month earlier than the National Resident Matching Program (NRMP).

Supply Projections. In 2008 in the United States there were 244 physicians in patient care per 100,000 people, and 314 total number of physicians per 100,000 people.[3] The Council on Graduate Medical

Education (COGME) forecasts a decrease to 301 total number of physicians per 100,000 in 2015. After that, the rate of population growth will continue to exceed the rate of growth in the number of physicians and a shortage of 85-96,000 physicians is predicted.[4] Even though the predicted shortage will affect every segment of the U.S. population, the most severe impact will be felt by the 20 percent of Americans who live in rural or inner-city locations designated as health professional shortage areas.

TASKS AND SUGGESTED TIMETABLE

The major impediment to decision making seems to be the lack of information that even fourth-year medical students have about themselves and the specialties. The ideal time to read this book is while you are still deciding whether to apply to medical school. Then you will be making a well-informed decision after considering what your future options might be. This does *not* mean that specialty choice should be decided prior to medical school admission. Medical students should know they will have to choose a specialty and be prepared to look for opportunities to compare their own preferences, interests, and talents with those of physicians practicing the various specialties. Primarily, medical students need to learn how to become good physicians, regardless of what specialties they will ultimately select.

Some of you may be reading this as first- or second-year medical students. You are probably starting to feel some apprehension about choosing a specialty and residency; yet there seems to be "plenty of time." At this early stage, the danger is in procrastinating. You should start today to attend seriously to this task, but pace yourself. At times you will feel motivated to think about your future plans; you will be particularly open to learning about the various specialties as you begin to work with clinical preceptors. You might wish to reread a pertinent chapter in this book as you start a new rotation; it may help you to understand the physician(s) you are working with and why you do or do not feel comfortable on the rotation.

The third year signals a time for at least deciding some basic likes and dislikes in medicine. You may want to find a "quick" answer to your specialty choice decision, but if you haven't done some prior preparation, you certainly won't be able to find the answer overnight. The best way to cope with your concerns about specialty choice at this stage is to tackle the problem a little bit each day, steadily building up your information resources. You cannot afford the luxury of waiting until you feel motivated—you need to do some work on self-assessment on a regular basis. This book can serve as a useful starting point.

The fourth year may bring doubts about your specialty decision. This experience is common to all who are making what they consider to be a "permanent" choice. A fourth-year student already interviewing for a residency position or even preparing to graduate, can still benefit from this book. You may be afraid that you have chosen the "wrong" specialty, and that is certainly understandable. If you truly have chosen a specialty that may not be satisfying to you, you will find out during your internship year. This book will help you understand that there is nothing "wrong" with you as a person if this happens, but rather that your talents, interests, and preferences would be better expressed in another area of medicine. Or you may pursue the specialty you have chosen, but consider the fact that you will be "different" from most of your colleagues in the field and you will develop your own area of interest within the specialty. Some specialties have typical "personalities" more than others, but all have practitioners who don't fit the stereotype. It is also possible for aspects of a specialty's activities to change. For example, with the introduction of fiberoptic endoscopy, gastroenterology became much more technologically oriented; it is now a procedure-based specialty with some similarities to surgery.

The reader who has already begun or is even finished training in a specialty might enjoy finding out that "the right choice" was made after learning about the practices of colleagues in other specialties. If you think that the other physician has an "easier" life, it might help to read what those in the specialty say. Or you may be contemplating a specialty change—to escape the feeling of being "trapped" in an area of medicine that no longer seems exciting. Be sure, however, that your expectations about another specialty are realistic.

The family members of the medical student or physician should be involved in the task of choosing a specialty and residency. It is very easy to feel excluded from the world of medicine with its unpronounceable words, closeness to issues of life and death, and seemingly endless demands. It is imperative for the physician to remember that he or she is a person first, one whose relationships with family or friends will have a profound impact on the medical practice, regardless of the specialty chosen. Ideally, both spheres of your world—your personal life and your professional life—will be thoughtfully considered and successfully pursued.

REFERENCES

1. Kendall PL. Medical specialization: Trends and contributing factors. In: Coombs RH, Vincent CE (eds). *Psychosocial aspects of medical training.* Springfield, IL: Charles C Thomas, 1971, p. 479.

2. Brotherton SE, Etzel SI. *Graduate medical education, 2010-11.* Appendix II, Table 1. *JAMA* 2011; 306(9):1015.

3. Physician Characteristics and Distribution in the U.S., 2010 edition. Division of Survey and Data Resources, American Medical Association, p. 437.

4. Council on Graduate Medical Education, Sixteenth Report, Physician Workforce Policy Guidelines for the United States, 2000-2020. Health Resources and Services Administration, U.S. Department of Health and Human Services. January 2005. p. xv.

Tasks and Suggested Timetable

Premedical School Years

1. Find out all you can about the career opportunities in medicine. Resources used and when: _____

2. Talk with physicians, residents, and medical students about their perceptions of medicine and how they impact on their personal lives.

   Name:_____Date:_____
   Comments: _____
   Name:_____Date:_____
   Comments:_____

3. If possible, get some practical volunteer or work experience in a hospital or health care setting.

   Experience: _____
   _____

4. Carefully consider your decision to apply for admission to medical school. Is a medical career right for you and are you choosing it for the right reasons?

First Year of Medical School

1. As you enter medical school, start a journal related to medical specialty choice. Write about classroom experiences that interest you (for career, research, further study), your impressions of clinical medicine (if offered in the first-year curriculum), and names of people you would like to get to know better.

   Start now by indicating the areas of medicine that interest you: __
   _____
   _____

   What do you hope to be doing ten years from now? _____
   _____
   _____

In what setting – rural or urban private practice, hospital based, academic, international, military - do you hope to spend your medical career?_____

_____

_____

2. Seek out a spectrum of "advisors" at your medical school—faculty physicians; residents; second- third-, and fourth-year medical students—and ask questions about their specialty interests.

Names of "advisors" and telephone numbers: _____

_____

_____

_____

3. Take advantage of any opportunity to observe physicians at work—during vacations in your hometown or weekend hospital rounds with a community or faculty physician.

Observation of: _____

_____

Date: _____ Comments: _____

_____

_____

_____

Observation of: _____

_____

Date: _____ Comments: _____

_____

_____

_____

4. Participate in extracurricular activities that may offer experience with medical care in the community, such as volunteering in a community-based free clinic or participating in a health fair.

Activities and dates: _____

_____

_____

_____

5. Pay attention to grades, especially those in the major clinical rotations; they *will* matter if you wish to enter the most competitive specialties.

6. Log into the Association of American Medical Colleges' Careers in Medicine website and complete the questionnaires in the self-assessment link.

7. Plan your summer activity early. Write your Curriculum Vitae for your applications if you are applying to competitive clinical or research programs.

The Summer Between the First and Second Year of Medical School

1. Based on your individual economic and/or emotional needs, you may work in a medical or nonmedical setting, or "take the summer off." Be aware that some residency programs will only invite you for an interview if you have done research in the specialty and this may be your only unscheduled time to do so. Research positions are generally available at your medical school—if you apply early enough in your first year—and they do pay a modest salary.

   My plans for the summer: _____

   _____

   _____

   _____

2. Spend time doing some serious self-assessment: Review your notes from your journal and clarify questions you have thought of in your first year by talking with physicians in various specialties and of various ages.

   Physicians contacted: _____

   _____

   _____

Comments: _____

_____

_____

_____

_____

3. Read about health care issues, such as cost containment, workforce debates, and ethical dilemmas in your local newspaper and national news magazines. Become a student member of a professional organization such as the American Medical Association, and receive the *Journal of the American Medical Association* and the *American Medical News,* both excellent resources on current health care issues.

   Issues and most interesting resources:

a. _____

b. _____

c. _____

4. Listen to what family members and friends are saying about your future career plans in medicine.

   What is my spouse/significant other saying? _____

   _____

   _____

   What are my friends/classmates saying? _____

   _____

   _____

Second Year of Medical School

1. Continue exploring various specialty areas by cultivating relationships with at least two mentors, individuals who will take a professional interest in you and offer nonjudgmental advice. Request a meeting in their offices; accept any opportunity to share in their family/community life.

   Name and telephone number: _____

   _____

Name and telephone number: _____

2. Write in your journal your impressions of clinical experiences, not just what you like or dislike, but why. Be specific about your patients, the problems faced and your feelings.

   My best experience was: _____

   _____

   _____

   Why? _____

   _____

   _____

   My worst experience was: _____

   _____

   _____

   Why? _____

   _____

   _____

3. Continue to pay attention to grades. Step 1 of the U.S. Medical Licensing Examination (USMLE) may be taken at the end of your second year. Residency programs weight these and Step 2 USMLE scores heavily in their consideration of applicants.

4. Ask faculty in your areas of specialty interest about clerkships or electives at other medical schools or internationally.

Electives Suggested	By Whom?	Why?
a._____	_____	_____
b._____	_____	_____
c._____	_____	_____
d._____	_____	_____

5. Read at least one book on specialty choice. Book(s) read: _____

   _____

   _____

   _____

6.   Career choices that interest you at this time and why: _____

_____

_____

Third Year of Medical School

1.   As you start your required clerkships, your journal will play a more important role by enabling you to review your notes a month or two later while on another service and cannot remember your specific feelings about a previous experience. Be sure to include positive and negative aspects of each clerkship, seeking insight as to why you feel the way you do about each field.

Clerkship I enjoyed most and why? _____

_____

_____

Clerkship I enjoyed least and why? _____

_____

_____

2.   When you find an especially satisfying clerkship, request a letter of reference for your residency applications. Even though it may seem early, it is important to have the letter written while all the details of your outstanding performance can be remembered. Letter requested, date and from whom? _____

_____

_____

Letter requested, date and from whom? _____

_____

_____

3.   Prepare a curriculum vitae to be used for residency applications. Date completed: _____

4.   Attend programs on specialty choice and residency planning offered by your medical school or a local, regional, or national student organization-sponsored program. Programs Attended_____ Date_____

5. At the end of your third year, review residency programs through the American Medical Association's computer directory titled the Fellowship and Residency Electronic Interactive Database Access System (AMA-FREIDA). Review web sites of those residency programs of greatest interest to you.

6. Continue talking to fourth year students, residents and faculty physicians about specialty options and specific programs.
    List of people talked to:

    Name   Specialty   Date

    _____   _____   _____

    _____   _____   _____

    _____   _____   _____

7. Write your personal statement for your applications.
    Date completed: _____

Fourth Year of Medical School

1. Sign the agreement with the NRMP (or other application service).
    Date done: _____

2. Make sure your have letters of recommendation being written. Make sure those writing have a copy of your curriculum vitae. Some residencies require a letter of recommendation from the chairperson (or official designee) of the department of your chosen specialty. Allow at least a month for preparation of these letters.

    Letter Requested From   Date

    _____   _____

    _____   _____

    _____   _____

    Review your Medical School Performance Evaluation (MSPE):

    _____

3. Take photographs for application forms.

4. Apply to Electronic Residency Application Service (ERAS) or other application service as early as possible. Date application submitted: _____

5. When invited for interviews, schedule them as early as possible.
6. Rank order programs before the deadline.
    Date Completed: _____
7. Match Day is in mid-March for programs in the National Resident Matching Program; earlier for other matching programs.

Copy and Place on Your Bulletin Board

Summary Checklist

___Meet at least three physicians practicing in a community setting. Talk with them about their practices and their lives.

___Get involved in at least one health-related community service activity, for example, with an indigent care clinic, health fair, or school health program.

___Participate in at least one medical student organization (AMSA, a specialty Interest Group, student government, etc.) to learn leadership and organizational skills.

___Find at least one mentor—someone who will take a professional interest in you and offer nonjudgmental advice.

___Go on website for information about specialty organization(s) of interest.

___Do a required or elective clerkship or preceptorship in your chosen field.

___Meet and talk with the chairperson (or the official designee) of the department of your chosen specialty and ask him/her for a letter of recommendation for residency applications.

___Request a letter of recommendation for residency applications from at least one physician in your chosen field.

___Read at least one book on specialty choice.

Finding A Specialty
That Is Right For You

Ask yourself the following questions *before* reading further in this book:
What are your top three personal and career goals?

1. _____

   _____

2. _____

   _____

3. _____

   _____

What role does work play in your life?_____

_____

_____

What are the characteristics of the medical specialties you might be
considering?_____

_____

Specialty   Characteristics

_____   _____

_____   _____

_____   _____

Are you able to correlate your abilities with the characteristics of the
various specialists? For example, how much are you energized by

people? Or are your "batteries" recharged by having some time alone? Some specialties, such as emergency medicine, require interaction with a multitude of people with a variety of problems in a relatively short period of time; other specialties, such as anesthesiology, involve a more focused interaction with one person for a longer period of time.

Even though your natural tendency is to want to start reading immediately about the specialties, it is important to understand the factors influencing your specialty preference. One of the major steps in the specialty selection process is knowing what questions to ask and when to ask them (see the selection questions below). Mary Lou Yates, MS, a career counselor in Davis, California, worked with me to identify five sequential stages in this process, with accompanying questions. It would be helpful if you and a family member or friend both answer them and then compare responses. It is very important to have feedback in this process. Sometimes, someone close to you may be more objective in assessing you than you can be.

Complete and Discuss with Those Closest to You

Stage 1

Information and Awareness—To assist you in selecting a major area of medicine, i.e., primary care versus tertiary care.

Why did I choose medicine as a career?

How did I make the decision to apply to medical school?

Do I have a special area of interest in medicine?

What do I know about the various specialties?

What are my family, friends, and faculty advising me to do?

Where do I want to live? Do I have geographic preferences/ restrictions?

Stage 2

Self-assessment—To assist you in discovering your values, needs, preferences.

What gives me the greatest energy?

What seems to drain my energy?

What two or three accomplishments have given me the most satisfaction?

Why did they seem satisfying?

What do I consider to be my greatest strengths?

What are my limitations?

Who has been a key mentor or role model for me? Why?

Stage 3

Career Exploration—To assist you in understanding how your values parallel what physicians do.

How would I describe my ideal daily work activities?

What patient age would I prefer to work with?

What kind of relationship do I want to have with my patients?

Do I want to work with a variety of common medical problems or singular, specialized problems?

Would I rather be the coordinator of care or the expert others use for referral?

How high is my tolerance level for undiagnosed problems and multiple symptoms?

Stage 4

Career Objectives—To assist you in setting goals and specific objectives.

What kind of lifestyle do I expect as a physician?

How much do I need to earn when I begin practice?

Describe the ideal practice setting.

What do I want from my career and how will I know when I achieve it?

What goals, other than career goals, have I set for myself for the next five years? For the next ten years?

How do I define success?

Stage 5

Residency Preparation—To assist you with decisions about electives, residency programs.

What is my choice of specialty?

What can I offer to my chosen specialty?

What concerns do I have about the specialty I am choosing?

What kinds of hands-on clinical experience have I had to confirm my career decision? What more do I need?

What criteria am I using to evaluate residency programs?

What are my family and friends saying about residency programs?

What can I offer to a residency that will make me the best possible candidate?

Factors in Specialty Choice

What influences your final choice of a specialty? There seems to be a combination of personal and societal factors involved. Sex, age, marital status, and geographic background all have been correlated with specialty choice. More than half the residents in dermatology, family medicine, obstetrics-gynecology, pediatrics, and psychiatry are women; more than half of the residents in anesthesiology, emergency medicine, orthopaedic surgery, radiology, thoracic surgery and urology are male.[1] Older and married students, especially those who grew up in a small town, are more likely to choose primary care specialties than their younger, single classmates from an urban background.[2,3] Other important factors are personality, life situation, initial perceptions of the various specialties, and medical school exposure to the specialties.

Personality. There is a place in medicine for all personality types. Medicine offers more choices in types of activities, work settings, interactions with people, and expression of personal values than any other profession.

Your own personality makeup will have a profound influence on your specialty choice. In addition to identifying and evaluating your goals, talents, and abilities, you need to match your own personal values and preferences to the specialty's requirements and characteristics. (The exercises at the end of each specialty chapter in Part 2 will assist you in this task.)

Medical students often embark on a frantic search for the one right specialty that will give them satisfaction, and are frustrated to find that they like bits and pieces of many specialties. If this is happening to you, it might be helpful to understand that you would most likely be happy in any of a number of fields. Different aspects of your personality will find satisfaction in more than one field—those who enjoy a long-term relationship with people will find such relationships in general pediatrics, general internal medicine, and family medicine; those who need immediate tangible results from their work will experience it in any of the surgical fields, dermatology, and anesthesiology; those who wish to affect changes for the future may find fulfillment in research in any specialty, in a public health career, or a focus on prevention in a clinical practice. As you become more aware of what gives you satisfaction and a sense of purpose and fulfillment, you will start to make some discoveries: You may prefer a fast-paced environment with a variety of activities and be attracted to both family medicine and emergency medicine, but if you need to know what happens to patients after you see them, family medicine might be more satisfying. You might prefer to work alone or in one-to-one relationships in a slower-paced setting and be drawn to both pathology and psychiatry, but if you need closure to problems, you'll find more satisfaction in pathology. Surgeons and psychiatrists are considered to be most consistent with the personality traits ascribed to them: Individuals who prefer surgery are usually decisive, practical, and dominant; those who prefer psychiatry are usually inquisitive, empathic, and low-key.

Resources to help learn more about yourself are available. Formal, standardized tests, such as the Myers-Briggs Type Indicator or the Medical Specialty Preference Inventory will show how your interests compare to those of physicians in the various medical specialties. Since these are self-report tests, their accuracy is dependent on your self-awareness and truthfulness. I have used the Myers-Briggs Type Indicator for twenty-five years and have found it to be helpful in discussing specialty choices with medical students. Kenneth Iserson's book[4] offers a Personal Trait Analysis. The Association of American Medical Colleges (AAMC) Careers in Medicine program on the website www.aamc.org/cim is designed to "develop strategies, materials, and real-time data to assist students with the process of career planning." It uses the techniques that I have recommended in past editions of this book and that I continue to advise for specialty choice: self-assessment, career exploration, decision making, and implementation throughout the entire four years of medical school.

Life Situation. There is a wide diversity of ages and life experiences among medical students today. Of graduating students in 2011 fifty percent are women; 28 percent, minorities; 16.3 percent, over the age of 30.[5]

Upon graduating from medical school, most students plan to enter clinical practice after residency training, either private or salaried. Of these, the majority plan to join a private clinical practice in a group of three or more physicians (22 percent). A substantial number (36 percent) plan to join a university faculty full time doing clinical or basic science teaching. Less than 10 percent plan to practice in a rural location.[5]

Studies have examined the relationship of debt and specialty choice, but the results have been contradictory. At graduation in 2011, eighty-four percent of graduating medical students have incurred educational debt, with the average amount of $160,911 (both educational and non-educational debt). Fifty percent have a debt of over $150,000.[5] Your financial indebtedness may be an important factor in your specialty choice decision if you feel increasing pressure to enter a field that you believe will allow a prompt repayment of your loan. It is advisable to consider, however, that there are an increasing number of programs designed to assist you in repaying your debt and, after the money is repaid, you will be practicing the specialty you chose for a long time.

Your relationship with a spouse or significant other may affect your specialty choice, particularly if two careers need to be co-ordinated, either geographically or in terms of time commitment. Medical students have indicated in surveys that lifestyle issues are a major factor in choosing a specialty. In the survey commissioned by Glaxo, Inc.[7] 81 percent of the 300 respondents cited "time for family" as one of the leading influences; only 33 percent named monetary considerations. Another report[8] of 346 students in nine medical schools found "perceived life-style," which included remuneration and prestige as well as personal time, to be most associated with choice of specialty. Schwartz et al[9] have classified specialties into two groups: those having a noncontrollable lifestyle and those with a controllable lifestyle. They defined "controllable lifestyle" specialties as those allowing the physician "control of work hours," and included in this group anesthesiology, dermatology, emergency medicine, neurology, ophthalmology, otolaryngology, pathology, psychiatry, and radiology. Physician contributors to this book, however, cite nighttime and weekend work, especially as the new member of a practice or salaried group, in many of the above specialties.

Therefore, I want to emphasize the following very strongly: YOU CAN WORK 24 HOURS A DAY IN WHATEVER SPECIALTY YOU CHOOSE. Medicine is very seductive and the emotional gratification can be enormous. Medicine is also a perfect escape from family responsibilities—you will not be criticized if you heed your beeper or page. No one will think badly of a physician who answers a call, even if it means missing a child's birthday party or the airplane to a vacation site—no one, that is, except family members who may suspect that coverage could have been arranged and patients reassured that competent care was available from another physician. It may be very hard for you to admit that you "need to be needed" by patients and that no matter what specialty you choose, this may become a pattern in your life.

There is one clear exception: The solo physician in a rural community will not be able to be "off call" unless coverage is arranged with another physician. Educating people about when a physician's expertise is necessary will be helpful in allowing the physician some personal time, but the services of a physician who chooses to practice in a remote or underserved area will be in great demand. You may see this as a fair tradeoff for the perceived benefits, such as living in a rural setting or having support from a small community. The solution to this situation, of course, is to have more physicians choose to practice in rural or inner-city underserved locations. Unfortunately, this does not seem to be the current trend, with only 30.7 percent of respondents to the 2011 AAMC Medical School Graduation Questionnaire[5] indicating interest in practicing in an underserved location.

The desire for a "controllable lifestyle" is also reflected by the movement to limit residents' working hours and the preference shift of physicians from private, fee-for-service practice to salaried positions with Health Maintenance Organizations (HMO) or group affiliation. In a survey of third-year residents[10] the majority, 37 percent, expect to work from 50 to 60 hours per week. In mid-life career shifts, physicians have traditionally favored specialties with more predictable work schedules, such as emergency medicine.[11]

Initial Perceptions of Various Specialties. Perceptions of a specialty may be influenced by past experiences. AAMC data[6] show that a decreasing number of medical students decided to be physicians before high school. In 2010, fifty-one percent of entering students reported that they decided to pursue a career as a physician during or after college. [6] Your career goal may be related to an illness you or a family member have experienced, which created an interest in helping people with a similar problem. Or you may feel "called" to follow in the steps of your hometown physician. You may have had a prior career in a health-related field or have participated in scientific research after college. Or, you may feel that the work you initially chose as a career did not bring the satisfaction you expected. Most commonly, I have found that the applicants to medical school I interview who have had careers in other fields miss the satisfaction of "making a difference in the lives of others" and are seeking more meaningful relationships in their work.17.7

Students have positive perceptions of some specialties when entering medical school. Childhood role models and personal experiences make family medicine appealing. The power of surgery, plus the image of surgeons, attracts some. Those with an early interest in pediatrics often have an affinity for children. Psychiatry attracts those who have a desire to learn more about human behavior. Obstetrics-gynecology interest is closely related to advocacy for women. In the 2010 AAMC Matriculating Student Survey Report[6], 17.7 percent of the entering students were planning to choose internal medicine; 13.7 percent, pediatrics; 10.2 percent, surgery; 8.7 percent, orthopaedic surgery; and 8.5 percent, family medicine.

Medical School Exposure to the Medical Specialties. Experiences in medical school, especially the 4 to 12 weeks spent on a clinical clerkship, can be positive or negative influences. You may have always wanted to be a surgeon but find that the reality of the operating room and postoperative care are quite different than you imagined. Or the personalities of the surgeons you work with do not seem to be compatible with yours. Your good performance on a clerkship will be a powerful affirmation of your abilities in that specialty; negative evaluations will probably cause you to question your interest and aptitude in that area of medicine.

You will undoubtedly be influenced by the opinions of your classmates as they discuss the various specialties' perceived status, potential for high income, and imagined physician lifestyle.

A physician on one of the clerkships may become a strong role model as you aspire to be "just like him or her." This can be an inspiration; it can also be dangerous if the role model does not exemplify his or her specialty peers.

Your school may have certain clinical departments that are stronger than others, and this can affect your specialty choice. State-supported schools graduate more students who choose primary care than private schools. Whether this is a result of admissions' policies and type of applicant or medical school experiences is unknown.

Medical school experiences alone, however, do not offer a balanced view of the specialty, and you need to seek out nonacademic contacts in the field of your choosing before making a final commitment. Students often are encouraged to "get a mentor," which may prove difficult if not pursued with knowledge and diligence. The following are some guidelines for selecting a mentor.

1. Decide on your career goals as realistically as you can. Then identify someone who is doing what you think you would like to do. Try to do this as early as possible, even in your first year of medical school. You could ask for suggestions from other students

or contact the specialty department administrator who usually has contact with students. If you would like a mentor who is in community practice, you could telephone your local medical society executive director for suggestions or ask for names of volunteer faculty from the specialty department. The Alumni Association of your school is another potential resource.

2.   Make an appointment to talk to your prospective mentor when you both have time for discussion (a 20- to 30-minute appointment is appropriate). To start off, you might ask the questions that are asked of respondents in Part 2 of this book—for example, "Why did you choose your specialty?" "What do you enjoy most about it?" "What advice would you give me since I'm interested in this specialty too?"

3.   Take time to develop the relationship. Both of you need to get to know each other and it would be helpful if you could get together in nonmedical as well as medical settings. You could invite your mentor to a sports game or to lunch, or to some other social activity. You might also offer to accompany him or her to hospital committee meetings or a community service club meeting.

4.   It will be very flattering for your mentor to know that you look to him or her for guidance, but don't become too dependent.

5.   More than one mentor is appropriate since it is helpful to have other opinions and advice. If you are interested in multiple specialties, then you definitely need to find additional mentors. Most physicians will be happy to continue to have a relationship with you even if you decide not to choose their specialties, but be aware that some may feel hurt and rejected. Clues as to their attitudes toward other specialties should be obvious early in your relationship. It would be best to find someone who respects all medical specialties as valuable and important and who will, therefore, respect your career interests if they turn out to be in a different specialty.

REFERENCES

1. Brotherton SE, Etzel, SI. Graduate medical education, 2010-11. Appendix II. Table 2. *JAMA* 2011: 306; (9):106-1017.

2. Davis WK, Coles C, Bouhuijs PAJ, Donaldson M, Dauphinee WD, Hoftvedt BO, McAvoy PA et al. Medical career choice: Current status of research literature. *Teaching and Learning in Medicine* 1990;2(3):130–138.

3. Xu G, Veloski JJ, Barzansky B. Comparisons between older and usual-aged medical school graduates on the factors influencing their choices of primary care specialties. *Acad Med* 1997;72(11):1003–1007.

4. Iserson K. Getting into a residency, 7th edition. Tucson: Galen Press, Ltd., 2008.

5. 2011 Medical School Graduation Questionnaire. Washington, DC: Association of American Medical Colleges.

6. The Section for Student Programs. 2010 Matriculating Student Survey Report. Washington, DC: Association of American Medical Colleges.

7. Medical students rate family over income in choosing specialty. *Physician's Financial News* 1988;6(1):1.

8. Schwartz RW, Haley JV, Williams C, Jarecky RK, Strodel WE, Young B, Griffin WO. The controllable lifestyle factor and students' attitudes about specialty selection. *Acad Med* 1990;65(3):207–210.

9. Schwartz RW, Jarecky RK, Strodel WE, Haley JV, Young B, Griffen WO. Controllable lifestyle: A new factor in career choice by medical students. *Acad Med* 1989;64(10):606–609.

10. Barnett B. Medical residents know their value. *Group Pract Jour* 1991;40(5):39.

11. Page L. Residency trend: Short hours, long money. *Amer Med News* 1990;33(43):3,43.

Considering Your Options

YOU NEED TO HAVE A CLEAR IDEA OF THE OPPORTUNITIES
available to you in medicine—whether you are going to pursue a
primary care specialty; be a referral physician; or use your specialty
training as a springboard to other endeavors either within or outside
of medicine, such as teaching, public service, or consulting with
private companies. Your medical school's resources may range from
a disorganized pile of papers and booklets in the office of the student
affairs dean to a medical specialty choice counseling program offering
workshops, administration of the Myers-Briggs Type Indicator or
other assessment instrument with personal consultation on results, and
community preceptorship experiences. Prior to the demise of the mandatory rotating internship, this task of educating about specialties was
considered unnecessary because the one-year internship experience
allowed exposure to the various specialties, at least in theory. In addition, male physicians were obliged to serve two years in the military,
further increasing their knowledge and experience base.

Even some fourth-year medical students are still unsure what specialty field they will enter. Most say that they do not have enough first-
hand experience in or knowledge of their various choices and, under
the present system of medical education, they never will. Therefore,
you need to gather information about the specialties and confirm that
those that interest you meet your personal needs and aspirations. There

are various ways of categorizing the specialties—generalist versus specialist; primary, secondary, and tertiary care; first-contact versus referral based. Each category has its own characteristics and you need to assess the appeal each has for you in an effort to start narrowing your choices.

Generalist vs. Specialist

A physician can be licensed to practice clinical medicine after one year of training in an approved residency program, but few students select this option. More than 98 percent of graduating U.S. medical students enter a residency program and 99 percent of these plan to complete at least three years of postgraduate training. Those who do not pursue postgraduate residency training right after graduation may be interested in a research career or may be taking time off with plans to continue their training later. Technically, all physicians who complete a residency training program are specialists in their medical fields.

Table 1: Characteristics of Generalists versus Specialists

Generalists	Specialists
Like working with people	Like taking care of people
Like variety in work activities	Prefer a narrower scope of professional activities
Have a higher tolerance for undiagnosed multiple symptoms	Satisfaction comes from action-oriented problems and curative intervention
Want to be involved in patients' lives	Prefer less involvement in patients' lives on a continuing basis

The words *generalists* and *specialists* are often used to identify those physicians who see a variety of patient problems versus those who only care for a specific area of medicine. For example, a family physician is called a generalist, while an ophthalmologist, whose training is limited to the care of eye problems, is termed a specialist. The generalist and the specialist have characteristic tendencies that will vary in strength in each individual; both may say that they like "variety" in their work, but the generalist will define variety to include not just types of medical problems, but also patients of various ages and both sexes. Family medicine would be the specialty with potentially the most variety; colon and rectal surgery with significantly less. Table 1 compares some characteristics of generalists and specialists.

Primary Care Specialties. Generalists are physicians in one of the three primary care specialties: family medicine, general internal medicine, and general pediatrics. There is ongoing debate as to whether obstetrics and gynecology should be classified as a primary care specialty. Generalists all have the characteristics of accessibility, accountability, comprehensiveness, continuity, and coordination shown in Table 2. Today, economic forces are adding cost-containment to this list.

Table 2: Characteristics of Primary Care Specialists

First contact care

Longitudinal responsibility

Small population served

Broad focus of care

Common problems

Integrationist approach

Community-based practice

Basic technology

Students entering medical schools express interest in family medicine and pediatrics to a higher degree than internal medicine, which is "discovered" by students after they enter medical school. The Centers for Disease Control reports that approximately one-quarter of all patient visits are to family physicians and one-third are to other primary care physicians – internists, pediatricians and obstetricians and gynecologists.[1] Most general internists and general pediatricians practice in large metropolitan areas. Family physicians are found in all settings, but they are the predominant physician providers in nonmetropolitan areas.

You may be interested in all three primary care specialties and find it difficult to decide on one of the three. The decision is often made on the basis of how willing you are to give up care of children or care of adults. Those who are more interested in either children or adults tend to choose pediatrics or internal medicine. Those who want the option of working with all ages in the broadest possible manner choose family medicine.

This comprehensiveness, however, may be intimidating to you, especially when most of your time in medical school is spent in a hospital setting with subspecialist role models who have a different level of need for closure and control of a situation than primary care physicians. However, even they do not know everything about their area of subspecialization. It is most important that you find your own personal comfort level in relationship to narrowing your focus.

Another characteristic of primary care involves becoming "part of the family." A revealing question to ask yourself is: How comfortable would I be to have my name and telephone number listed next to those of relatives, the religious advisor, and others important in the lives of the family members? A primary care physician will often be accorded a place in the family's life that may be either gratifying or uncomfortable for you.

Finally, by being the physician of first contact, there will be more uncertainty involved in patient care. The diagnosis or problem will not always be immediately evident and your tolerance for ambiguity will be a factor in your comfort level.

Secondary Care Specialties. Specialists can be divided into secondary and tertiary care physicians. Both share the characteristics of being "experts" in a particular area of medicine. Examples of secondary care specialists are general surgeons who operate to remove an acute appendix; the internal medicine and pediatric subspecialists who will offer opinions on further medical care of complicated problems; and psychiatrists who will provide ongoing therapy for a mentally ill patient. Sometimes included in this category are obstetricians/gynecologists who in urban settings may be the primary care providers for women. Similarly, emergency medicine physicians are also providing primary care to a large segment of the population in urban hospitals. The characteristics of secondary care specialties are outlined in Table 3.

Table 3: Characteristics of Secondary Care Specialties

Based on referral

Intermediate focus of care

Uncommon problems

Episodic care

Intermediate size population served

Hospital based practice

Consultant approach

Complex technology

Primary care physicians refer patients to secondary care specialists for consultation when there are health care needs that the primary care physician chooses not to offer in his or her practice. A physician's license is granted to practice medicine and surgery, and restrictions are individually selected. Physicians serving in rural or underserved areas of the world may include all medical and surgical services possible in their practices—if they don't help the patient, there is no one else to do so. Only by leaving their geographic area would a patient be able to have the services of a secondary care specialist.

In areas where there are a variety of health care professionals, it is expected that physicians will be granted hospital privileges and will offer services in areas of medicine and surgery that reflect their training and continued expertise. A surgeon would seek consultation from a patient's family physician concerning medical problems and history; a family physician would seek psychiatric opinion on a delusional schizophrenic patient. There are certain societal expectations involved in this process—a geriatric patient would be surprised to be referred to a pediatrician; a pregnant woman would not want to have an orthopaedic surgeon provide her ongoing prenatal care.

Tertiary Care Specialties. A primary care physician may refer directly to a tertiary care specialist who usually is located in a large referral center with teaching programs. A primary care physician may recommend that a patient see a tertiary care specialist for a specific treatment, such as a brain tumor requiring surgery. Tertiary care physicians tend to be involved in highly technological fields, such as thoracic surgery and nuclear medicine. Characteristics of tertiary care specialties are outlined in Table 4.

Table 4: Characteristics of Tertiary Care Specialties

Based on referral

Narrow focus of care

Large population served

Complex/rare problems

Discontinuous type of care

Medical center practice base

Referral approach

Innovative technology

Support Service Specialties. Some medical specialties are categorized as support services. This includes physicians who serve as consultants to other physicians, such as the pathologist or radiologist. Those who work in institutional settings, such as the occupational medicine physician, may be providing primary care when personally examining and treating company employees and support services when consulting with the personnel director on employee health benefits or supervising other physicians who provide direct care.

REFERENCE

1. Hsiao, CJ, Cherry DK, Beatty PC, Rechtsteiner EA. National Ambulatory Medical Care Survey: 2007 Summary. National Health Statistics Reports. Number 27, November 3, 2010, p.2.

Deciding On A Specialty In An Uncertain World

"Will I be able to get a residency position in my chosen specialty?"

"Is there an oversupply, undersupply, or balance in specialties or is there a total oversupply of physicians in the United States?"

"After residency, and perhaps fellowship training, will I be able to find a job?"

"What about managed care? Should it be a determining factor in my specialty choice?"

These were student concerns for the fourth edition of this book nine years ago. Are they still the questions students are asking? I believe they are, but there is another question that I hear increasingly from students and needs to be addressed first:

"What do I do if I can't decide on a specialty by the beginning of my fourth year?"

The Undecided Student

This is a common question from those who counsel students at the medical schools: "I have a medical student starting his fourth year who is somewhat anxious regarding specialty selection. He has not done much to help himself make an informed decision, and, at this point is looking for direction."

At the Oregon Health & Science University School of Medicine there are photographs by class year of all the students on a board across the hallway from my office. Every June, I take down the graduating class pictures and make room for the incoming class in September. As part of this process I carefully cut out the pictures of those who have delayed graduation and tape their pictures to the new 4th year class roster. It no longer surprises me when I move 20 percent of the pictures to the new roster. In other medical schools the scenario might be that some students graduate, but delay starting a residency. Admittedly, most take time off saying they wish to pursue personal interests or to have an experience that work and family might preclude in the future. Or, might it be that they have not found their specialty role in medicine or that they feel they would be more competitive in their chosen field if they engage in research for an additional year before applying to residency? One estimate is that about 400 medical school graduates delay starting residency after graduation. [1] Some return to medicine; some do not.

I offer the reader a question and a few suggestions which may help you if you are undecided about your specialty choice late in your medical school years. The question is: "What did you imagine you would do in medicine when you applied to medical school?" Even though there is a widespread belief that students change their initial specialty choice, I believe that most student stay interested in the same "cluster" of specialties, e.g., primary care specialties, surgical specialties, non-direct patient care specialties, that were of interest when they entered medical school. If you are honest about your strengths and the reasons you applied to medical school, you will understand why you are attracted to certain specialties and not to others.

If you are truly struggling to find your direction in medicine, taking a year off during or after medical school may be an appropriate choice. My strong suggestion is to use the time wisely. If your inclination is to choose a clinical career, find a volunteer or paid position where you will gain experience working with the type of patient seen by physicians in the specialties you are considering. An international experience will give you exposure to a variety of clinical specialties as will working in a community clinic serving a low income population in the U.S. A year of doing research, working in an operating room, or serving at a local, state or federal public policy or legislative office might be just what you need to see your specialty choice in perspective.

You may be advised to graduate and take a transitional year of postgraduate training since it will allow you to experience a number of medical specialties. This course of action will keep you engaged in medical training and relieve your medical school of the burden of helping you with your residency match, especially if you leave the geographic area. But I do not think it is the best plan. Transitional postgraduate training has become very competitive since many students are applying for specialties that they match in a broad-based first year of training. If you do match in a transitional or preliminary year position, you will have to apply for a residency during your "internship" year when taking off time to interview may be problematic. You may need to repeat your "internship" year, which is not a pleasant prospect. If you take a transitional year, you will need to explain why you chose this path. This is not the best way to start your first year as a physician.

Workforce Projections

As much as I advise students to choose a specialty based on their own temperaments, talents, and satisfactions, it is difficult to ignore what is being said by classmates, physicians, and the media about today's medical marketplace. The cycle of "feast or famine" in the physician workforce gained attention in the 1960s when fear of a physician shortage resulted in a massive federal government program to establish new medical schools and hospitals. Enrollment in medical schools more than doubled in the 1970s. A warning of a coming physician surplus was sounded in 1980 by the Graduate Medical Education National Advisory Committee (GMENAC), the details of which I described in the first two editions of this book.

Why is a physician surplus such a concern? First, there is the expense of training physicians and the fear that they will not find employment in their chosen fields. However, a greater societal concern is the perception that the greater the number of physicians, the larger the amount of spending on medical care. Doctors are perceived as generating health care costs. After the GMENAC report, the federal government stopped offering financial incentives to increase the number and size of medical schools and enrollment stayed at approximately 16,000 students. However, the number of residents continued to rise from 61,819 in 1983 to 96,410 in 2001 as a result of continued federal funding to Graduate Medical Education (GME) and an influx of international medical school graduates to fill the residency positions available.[2]

Is there really a surplus or a shortage of physicians? It seems to depend upon whom you ask. Following years of studies and recommendations by individual researchers and national commissions, six of the nation's most prestigious medical organizations released a historic Consensus Statement on Physician Workforce on February 28, 1997 to guide the U.S. Congress in policy deliberations regarding the physician workforce. The Association of American Medical Colleges, American Association of Colleges of Osteopathic Medicine, American Medical Association, American Osteopathic Association, Association of Academic Health Centers, and the National Medical Association all agreed that "the current rate of physician supply (the number of physicians entering the workforce each year) is clearly excessive." The report continues, "To decrease the rate of physician supply, limits must be placed on the number of medical school graduates entering GME" and ". . . it is imperative that the federal government partner with the medical education community to achieve this goal."[3] Recommendations include the reduction of GME positions funded by the federal government to a number closer to the number of U.S. medical school graduates each year, but sufficient to allow all M.D. and D.O. graduates of accredited U.S. medical schools an opportunity to match in an accredited GME program. Other recommendations address narrowing the opportunities for foreign-born physicians who are graduates of non-U.S. medical schools, offering incentives to those interested in serving rural and inner city populations, advocating a new all-payer fund for GME support, supporting transitional funding for teaching hospitals willing to downsize their GME programs and a stable source of support for all teaching hospitals, and the establishment of a new workforce advisory group to oversee the process. Most of these recommendations were included in the Balanced Budget Act of 1997 or referred for study. One tangible outcome is the ruling that there will be a limit set for direct graduate medical education payment to hospitals based on the number of residents in the institution as of December 31, 1996. In effect, this means that the institution will not receive funding for additional positions after this date.[2]

One measurement of the physician workforce is the ratio of physicians per 100,000 population. In 1980 the ratio was 198; in 1990, it increased to 233; by 2000, it was 294.[4] Critics of this measurement maintain that it ignores specialty and geographic maldistribution as well as quality of care offered.[5]

An early study by Cooper [6] discounts a future national surplus of physicians, although it concedes that there are and will continue to be local and regional surpluses which will need "local solutions." More recent research by Cooper [7] concluded that there will be a deficit of 200,000 physicians by 2020 due to a reduction in physician work effort, the aging physician population, an underestimation of the growth of U.S. population, and an increase in non-physician providers.

Health maintenance organization (HMO) data have been used to forecast future workforce needs. Weiner[8] predicted an excess of 165,000 physicians by the year 2000, with the supply of generalists in balance but a 60 percent glut of specialists. Seventy percent of the HMO executives surveyed in a recent report from the Harvard School of Public Health[9] agreed that there are too many specialists. But 60 percent of the physician specialists surveyed responded that an excess in their fields does not exist, except in cardiology, dermatology, and gastroenterology. Of the primary care physicians surveyed, 70 percent believed that a surplus in their specialties does not exist.

To compound the issue, there are conflicting data from physician recruiters. One major recruiting company, Merritt, Hawkins & Associates, reported a surge of demand for radiologists, cardiologists, and orthopaedic and general surgeons between 2000-2001. However, physicians have seen these cycles in the past and say that they can be caused by various forces including emerging technology, societal concerns, changes in reimbursement systems and even the media. [10]

Students' Decisions

Are medical students making specialty choice decisions based on what they think the medical marketplace will need and financially support? Or are they following their "gut" feelings? Should you abandon your early interests in an area of medicine for which you have the most talent and skill? I have had surgeons tell me, "If I couldn't be a surgeon, I would not want to be in medicine." I don't believe that there is just one *right specialty* for each of you; you could probably be happy in more than one specialty. (Remember, surgical procedures are performed in many specialties, not just one.) But you also want to find satisfaction in what you do. Students are struggling with this balancing of needs.

To get some insight into this issue, I asked two questions of fourth year graduating students at the Oregon Health & Science University School of Medicine: " What specialty did you think you would choose when you applied to medical school?" and "If you are not entering that specialty, why did you change your plan?" The table on the following page lists answers from those who changed specialty interest.

Students who followed their original specialty choice were mostly those who had experience in the specialty prior to starting medical school. Those choosing family medicine cited the role models they had prior to medical schools as major influences in their decision as well as the breadth and variety of the specialty, the long term relationship with patients and families and the opportunity to work in a wide variety of settings. Also, following their initial interests were those choosing surgery, who felt they were "most satisfied" in the operating room and emergency medicine physicians who had worked in this setting before medical school.

Pre-medical School Interest	Specialty Choice	Reason for Change
General Surgery	Anesthesiology	Lifestyle during and after residency
Emergency Medicine	Internal Medicine, probably subspecialist	Realized in 3rd year that I wanted some relationships with patients and to be a specialist rather than a generalist. Also, more internal medicine residencies in same city as med school and my wife did not want to move.
Family Medicine	Orthopaedics	Operating was "exciting, uplifting and challenging."
		The camaraderie among the residents/physicians in orthopaedics, the grateful patients, and patients who value physical activity.
Family Medicine	Dermatology	Discomfort in third year family medicine clerkship with too much variety and the need for competence. Lifestyle issues.
Psychiatry	Family Medicine	Breadth and depth of care in personal relationships, variety, wanted medical aspects in practice
Internal Medicine/ Pediatrics/ Family Medicine	Internal Medicine	Wanted to involve patient in the treatment plan, work with adults to manage his or her own health care; too much to know in Family Medicine
Preventive Medicine/Primary Care	Pediatrics	Opportunity to pursue subspecialty – keeping options open
Orthopaedics/ Oncology	Radiation Oncology	Lifestyle, technology, didn't want to deal with medical issues
Obstetrics	Family Medicine	Couldn't give away the babies after birth; liked taking care of the whole family; obstetrics was too surgical
Anesthesiology (pre-med experience with anesthesiologist)	Surgery	Personality and values most consistent with surgeons; wanted to be "in charge"

Pre-medical School Interest	Specialty Choice	Reason for Change
Internal Medicine	Anesthesiology	Did not like outpatient medicine. Likes procedural nature of anesthesiology, the rapid feedback of labs and instrumentation, the life-and-death relevance to the work.
Family Medicine	Urology	Likes caring for people on shorter-term basis and having a more immediate impact on their health. Lifestyle issues.

As you read Parts 2 and 3 of the book, think about *why you came to medical school* and how you are *similar to or different from the physicians* in each of the specialties. After that, consider *where you will practice* as you read Part 4 of the book. And, finally, remember that whatever you choose as a specialty will be *your professional identity* and those in the field will be your colleagues.

Make your decisions based on who you are and what you dream to be rather than on economic projections and marketplace changes that may or may not happen. Jerome Kassirer[12] tells of a colleague who was asked to speculate how medical care would be organized five years hence. He summed up the status of predictions: he said he wasn't even sure what the system would be like when he got back to his office that afternoon.

REFERENCES

1. Ziegler J. Time out. *The New Physician* 2002;51(4):19-22.
2. Dunn MR, Miller RS, Richter TH. Graduate medical education, 1997–1998. *JAMA* 1998;280(9):809–812.
3. Consensus Statement on Physician Workforce. Revised December 29, 1997. From Internet http://www.aamc.org/meded/edres/workforc/start.htm.
4. Council on Graduate Medical Education. Third Report: Improving Access to Health Care Through Physician Workforce Reform:

Directions for the 21st Century. Rockville, MD: U.S. Department of Health and Human Services, 1992.

5. Petersdorf RG. Projections for the generalist physician. [Letters.] *JAMA* 1995; 274(23):1833–1834.

6. Cooper RA. Perspectives on the physician workforce to the year 2020. *JAMA* 1995; 274(19):1534–1543.

7. Cooper RA, Getzen TE, McKee HJ, Laud P. Economic and demographic trends signal an impending physician shortage. *Health Affairs* 2002; 21(1):140-154.

8. Weiner JP. Forecasting the effects of health reform on U.S. physician workforce requirement: Evidence from HMO staffing patterns. *JAMA* 1994;272:222–230.

9. Diogo S. HMO execs claim oversupply of doctors—but docs don't agree. *Amer Med News* 1998;41(33):9.

10. Ehmann LC. The ups and downs of physician compensation. Unique Opportunities 2002; 12(3):34-44.

11. Hawley C. Impact of managed care on medical students. *Hosp Pract* 1997;(2):187.

12. Kassirer J. Is managed care here to stay? *N Engl J Med* 1997;336(14):1014.

PART 2

THE SPECIALTIES
AND SUBSPECIALTIES

Allergy and Immunology

FAST FACTS:

Number of fellowship positions matched in 2010 to start in 2011 : 79

Competitiveness: Medium (80% of US grads matched); helpful to have research experience or a residency at a large academic center

Length of training: 5 years (2 years after 3 years of internal medicine or pediatrics residency)

Number of fellowship programs: 79

Number of fellows in training: 219

Number in US Board Certified in Allergy and Immunology: 608

Number Board Certified in 2009: 145; Number Recertified in 2009: 203

Starting median compensation: $135,000

Median compensation for all physicians in specialty: $183,000

Mean # of hours weekly in patient care activities: 35.3

Mean # of hours weekly in professional activities: 40.7

SOMETIMES CONSIDERED TO BE A SUBSPECIALTY OF BOTH internal medicine and pediatrics, allergy and immunology was given specialty status with the formation in 1972 of the American Board of Allergy and Immunology (ABAI).

The work of clinical allergists is more familiar to the public than the more scientifically oriented activities of the immunologist, but both allergy and immunology are concerned with the human body's reaction to foreign substances, no matter what the practice setting.

Fellowship Information. A two-year fellowship in allergy and immunology is available to those who have completed three years of training in either internal medicine or pediatrics. Training is in both pediatric and adult allergy and immunology and it is expected that at least 25 percent of the resident's two years will be spent in patient care activity. Active research is strongly encouraged.

Board Certification. The ABAI is a Conjoint Board of the American Board of Internal Medicine (ABIM) and the American Board of Pediatrics (ABP). You are required to have received board certification in either internal medicine or pediatrics and to have successfully completed at least two years of an approved training program in allergy and immunology prior to applying for board certification in allergy and immunology.

Certification of Added Qualification in Clinical and Laboratory Immunology is open to physicians certified by the American Board of Internal Medicine, the American Board of Pediatrics, or the American Board of Allergy and Immunology who have an additional year of training in allergy and immunology. Those physicians in charge of laboratories and/or who have prior training in rheumatology, nephrology, oncology, infectious diseases, or nuclear medicine are most likely to seek this certification.

Supply and Projections. The number of allergists/immunologists had slowly decreased over the years due to training numbers not keeping up with retirement rate of practicing A/I physicians. However, in 2000 there was a resurgence in training in the specialty. A 2006 report[1] concluded that there would be increased demand for allergy and immunology physicians driven by the increased volume of allergy and asthma related conditions and that a moderate shortage would exist in 2024.

Economic Status and Types of Practice. Income is highly variable depending on the type of practice. Salary levels in academic institutions, government agencies, and corporations are often less than earnings in private practices. The focus in the former is more on research, teaching, and administration rather than on clinical aspects.

Further Information. The American Academy of Allergy, Asthma, and Immunology, 555 East Wells Street, Suite 1100, Milwaukee, WI 53202. Telephone: (414) 272-6071. Internet address: www.aaaai.org.

The Academy sponsors the Chrysalis Project to encourage medical student interest in this specialty. Travel and housing grants to the national meeting, and mentoring opportunities are available. There is a Summer Fellowship Grant program to pursue research during the summer after the first year of medical school.

A COMPOSITE PICTURE OF THE ALLERGIST/ IMMUNOLOGIST

Why Choose Allergy and Immunology?

Initial attractions to this field included role models, a research interest, and a sense of being able to help people who are suffering. Almost all respondents had little knowledge of this specialty during medical school and made their career choice while in either a pediatric or internal medicine residency: "During residency, I worked with well-trained allergists in the care of severely asthmatic children."

Decisions to subspecialize were made because pediatrics and general internal medicine both were perceived as having too much night call, a high volume of patient demands causing physician "burnout," and low income. One respondent did not like the geriatric aspects of internal medicine.

Respondents reported various reasons for not wanting certain fields: surgery—"It's not for my personality type"; oncology—"there's too much death and little 'success' "; psychiatry—"there are no real cures"; obstetrics and gynecology—"erratic hours"; other specialties that are "psychologically draining." (Ed. note: The respondents say they would not enjoy specialties that do not have patient contact so it seems that they are interested in patient care, but not at an emotionally intense level.)

What Do You Like Most About Allergy and Immunology?

The greatest enjoyment comes from two sources: (1) the challenges—"the excitement of asking new questions and constantly learning new facts"; and (2) the success of patient care—"seeing patients 'turn around' who have previously been managed but were not doing well." In a career satisfaction study[2] data show that 48.2 percent are "very satisfied" with only 10.7 percent "dissatisfied" in this specialty.

What Do You Like Least About Allergy and Immunology?

Those who care for patients find it difficult to deal with patients who are "non-compliant and argumentative," have psychosomatic illnesses, and make "unnecessary telephone calls late at night." Those in more administrative positions dislike the paperwork and "being unable to fully manage or control day-to-day clinic functions and personnel." One respondent reported that subspecialization "limits the spectrum of diseases and increases the repetitive nature of medicine."

What Is Your Typical Daily Schedule?

Allergy and immunology is primarily a referral practice and hospital visits mostly are consultations at the request of other physicians. Some respondents would limit their clinical care to children, but most would care for both adults and children. In a private practice, much time (90 percent) may be spent in clinical care; in a research or academic setting, 100 percent of the time may be nonclinical. In a practice setting, work schedules usually are regular, but there may be emergency calls related to asthma attacks or severe allergic reactions during office hours and at night or on weekends.

What Abilities and Talents Are Important in Allergy and Immunology?

The emphasis will depend on the type of practice; those in a clinical setting need to develop good communication skills, that is, "the talent to teach and explain disease processes and the role of various types of treatment for these illnesses." Technically, you need to have the "ability to perform and interpret skin tests." Those working in a research setting need to have organizational skills—"the ability to manage and motivate others and to supervise a clinical lab."

What Personality Traits Characterize Allergists and Immunologists?

Regardless of practice setting, allergists and immunologists characterize themselves as "detectives," having the capacity to integrate and synthesize new and complex ideas. They are patient and compassionate, but not strongly oriented toward psychological areas. This specialty has a place for quite opposite personalities—those who are more comfortable in research activities and those who enjoy patient care.

What Advice Would You Give a Medical Student Interested in Allergy and Immunology?

As this specialty research expands, basic science and an understanding of immunology become increasingly more important. However, you are advised to get the best clinical training possible for a broad knowledge of medical science. One respondent advocated a fellowship program in allergy and immunology with a strong emphasis on pulmonary physiology.

What Are the Future Challenges to Allergy and Immunology?

The future research challenges and the need to find sources of funding for that research are closely related. There is an open field in the potential to gain a better understanding of disease mechanisms, improved therapeutics, and the development of immunotherapy.

There is concern about "some physicians becoming too dependent on tests as a means of diagnosing and treating allergies—all tests are just tests and need to be interpreted in light of the patient's history and account for only part of caring for the patient."

Respondents continue to discuss serious competition from other subspecialties that have developed similar interests in areas of allergy and immunology: rheumatologists in autoimmune disease, hematologists/oncologists in bone marrow transplantation, otolaryngologists in allergic rhinitis, and pulmonologists in asthma. However, with the projected workforce shortage in this and other specialties, this concern will diminish.

REFERENCES

1. Forecasting Allergy and Immunology Physician Supply and Demand through 2024. The Center for Health Workforce Studies, University at Albany, School of Public Health, Rensselaer, N.Y. June 2006. www.aaaai.org/members/resources/workforce/FinalSurveyReport.pdf accessed December 22, 2010.

2. Leigh JP,Kravitz RL, Schembri M, Samuels SJ, Mobley S. Physician career satisfaction across specialties. *Arch Intern Med* 2002;162:1577-1584.

Job Values Selection of Allergists and Immunologists

You can complete the questionnaires and obtain your scores for all specialties online at http://www.sdn.net, or compare your job values (as recorded in the Appendix) with the job values of allergy and immunology respondents on the next page.

Allergists' and Immunologists' Choices:	My Choices:
1. Working with my mind	1._____
2. Independence	2._____
2. Taking care of people	3._____
2. Variety	4._____
(there is a three-way tie for second place)	

No one chose: Feedback from others

Summary Profile of Allergists and Immunologists (derived from questionnaire answers)	**My Personal Profile as an Allergist and Immunologist**			
They tend to:	I tend to: (circle one number)			
	Never	Rarely	Sometimes	Frequently	Always
Ask why	1	2	3	4	5
Pay attention to details	1	2	3	4	5
Enjoy taking care of people	1	2	3	4	5
Become bored with repetitive activity	1	2	3	4	5
Value time off	1	2	3	4	5
Like complex problem solving	1	2	3	4	5
Need control over a situation	1	2	3	4	5
Value independence highly	1	2	3	4	5
Enjoy being an "expert"	1	2	3	4	5
Enjoy research	1	2	3	4	5

Add total of numbers circled to get your TOTAL SCORE:_____

Transfer score to the Appendix.

Allergy and immunology.

    sounds like me _____

    could be a possibility _____

    doesn't sound like me at all _____

Anesthesiology

FAST FACTS:

Number of first year positions offered in the NRMP in 2011 : 841
2011 US grad fill rate in the first year NRMP: 79.8%
Number of second year positions offered in the NRMP in 2011 : 563
2011 US grad fill rate in the second year NRMP: 76.6 %
Length of training: 4 years (including a Clinical Base (or PGY-1)) year
Number of residency programs: 102 have first year entry positions; 83 have second year entry positions
Number of residents in training: 5322
Competitiveness: High
Competitive applicants have: high grades in required clerkships, a high grade in elective in anesthesiology, high class rank.
US senior matched applicants' mean USMLE Step 1 score is: 224
US senior matched applicants' mean USMLE Step 2 CK score: 230
Number in US Board Certified in Anesthesiology: 28,969
Range of compensation: $274,000-$338,000
Average work hours per week: 61

MEDICAL STUDENTS ARE OFTEN UNAWARE OF THE ANESTHE-siologist's role until after they take a clinical rotation. Preclerkship descriptions of anesthesiologists as "high-class technicians" or

"Ph.D.-inclined people having more of an exact science approach than a clinical one" are in contrast to such postclerkship descriptions as "a real lifesaver" and the physician who practices "the most exact art in medicine."[1]

According to the American Board of Anesthesiology's definition of the specialty, the anesthesiologist performs a variety of activities: manages procedures for rendering a patient insensible to pain and emotional stress during surgical, obstetrical, and certain medical procedures; supports life functions under the stress of anesthetic and surgical manipulations; clinically manages the patient unconscious from whatever cause; manages problems in pain relief; manages problems in cardiac and respiratory resuscitation; applies specific methods of inhalation therapy; and clinically manages various fluid, electrolyte, and metabolic disturbances. Only two of the above strictly involve operating room activities. The anesthesiologist visits each patient preoperatively to evaluate the individual's readiness for surgery, discuss the procedures, and allay patient anxiety. In addition, the anesthesiologist is responsible for postanesthesia recovery room care.

Residency Information. In May 1985 the residency training program in anesthesiology increased from three to four years. The first year, the Clinical Base Year, is essentially an internship in a clinical specialty. Some programs will set up this year for you while others will require you to find your own. The next three years offer training in clinical anesthesia and critical care. You may choose to focus on obstetric, neurosurgical, cardiothoracic, pediatric, or ambulatory anesthesia, but only critical care, hospice and palliative care and pain management are formal subspecialties.

Board Certification. To be board certified you must successfully complete both written and oral examinations. Three years of clinical anesthesiology residency, including two months of pain management and two months of critical care experience, are required to be eligible for board certification. The American Board of Anesthesiology offers Certificates of Special Qualifications in Critical Care Medicine, Hospice and Palliative Care and Pain Medicine.

Supply and Projections. The number of anesthesiologists has almost tripled in the past 25 years. There are approximately 31,000 board-certified physicians in this field. Declining surgery rates and the use of certified registered nurse anesthetists (CRNAs) had led to fewer practice opportunities, especially for recent graduates in the mid and late 1990s. However, a growing demand for surgical care, large numbers of early physician retirements and a drastic reduction in the number of training positions a decade ago created the current shortage of anesthesiologists.

Economic Status and Types of Practice. Two decades ago, anesthesiology was at the top of the income data for physicians. Salaries decreased dramatically in the mid 1990s. Currently, due to a shortage of anesthesiologists, salaries are again rising. The latest data from a variety of national surveys report mean recruitment income offered as $274,000 - 338,000. [2]

Patients' charges are calculated according to various factors: nature and risks of the operation, amount of time spent, patient's health status, and whether the surgery is elective or emergency. As surgical cases become more complex, operations take longer. Also, hospitals customarily cover many practice expenses for the anesthesiologists on staff. Most anesthesiologists are engaged in group practice, either on a fee-for-service basis or on the hospital staff. You might develop a special interest in critical care, pain clinic work, or respiratory therapy.

Further Information. The American Society of Anesthesiologists, 520 N. Northwest Highway, Park Ridge, IL 60068. Telephone: (847) 825-5586. Internet address: www.asahq.org.

The American Osteopathic College of Anesthesiology, 17201 E. Hwy. 40, Suite 204, Independence, MO 64055. Telephone: (816) 373-4700.

The American Academy of Pain Medicine, 4700 W. Lake Avenue, Glenview, IL 60025. Telephone: (847) 375-4731. Internet address: www.painmed.org.

A COMPOSITE PICTURE OF THE ANESTHESIOLOGIST

Why Choose Anesthesiology?

The initial appeal of anesthesiology includes "patient contact but no long-term follow-up or responsibilities," "precision and practical aspects of the specialty," "action and excitement of the operating room," "acute nature of care," and the "variety of subspecialties" in the field. One respondent describes anesthesiology as the "bridge or link between basic sciences and clinical medicine."

Anesthesiologists would not want to practice specialties that they characterize as "not having enough action," having "oppressive hours," "dealing with psychosomatic problems," and/or having "patients with chronic diseases that you can't really help." Two respondents had considered surgery as a career choice but had not pursued it—one because of the prolonged training period, and the other because it was ". . . impossible for a woman to get a surgery residency in my day."

What Do You Like Most About Anesthesiology?

Although anesthesiology is thought to have little primary patient contact, the number one satisfaction reported by physician respondents involves the doctor/patient relationship—"allaying fear and anxiety in a very stressed group of human beings," "my supportive role relative to the patient." An obstetric anesthesiologist says, "I do primarily regional techniques so that my patients are not asleep and this allows for better contact with patients."

High on the list is the satisfaction from immediately seeing the results of one's efforts—"titrated patient care with rapid feedback is a way of life for an anesthesiologist"; "I enjoy the actual process of devising an anesthetic plan preoperatively, carrying that plan out, and being able to see the end results of the plan all within a 24-hour period"; "Things happen. You evaluate critical situations, make decisions, give drugs that produce immediate dramatic changes."

What Do You Like Least About Anesthesiology?

Issues concerning control over time are cited, with night call the least liked aspect of the work. Other time-related problems are "the frustrations of scheduling, of coordinating with other anesthesiologists, surgeons, operating room time, operating room nurses." One respondent says, "the lack of control over hours, patients, personnel with whom one works"; another answers, "You can't produce results independently of others. It is hard to be better than the "team" on which you are playing."

Surgeons come in for various levels of criticism: "It is often unpleasant to have to run the operating room and deal with capricious, self-centered individuals such as most surgeons"; "Having to work with egotistical, immature, disorganized, slow surgeons is number one"; "A few surgeons are difficult to work with."

The lack of public and medical professional appreciation and recognition is also unappealing.

What Is Your Typical Daily Schedule?

The working day ranges from 8 to 12 hours. Anesthesiologists start early, arriving at the hospital at 7:00 AM. Depending on the setting, activities vary: Those in private and hospital-based practices are in the operating room most of the day and then make pre- and postoperative rounds in the late afternoon; those in academic settings engage in educational conferences, research and writing activities, administrative meetings, and teach residents and nurses in addition to operating room duties. A few respondents report no true lunch hour, "only a sandwich between cases."

Anesthesiologists in private practice describe being "on call" as often as every fifth night at which times they are up much of the night with mostly obstetric and emergency operations. Academicians report "on call" duties two or three nights a month and one to two weekend days per month; they also have to be available during the entire night "on call" to discuss cases and supervise residents' work. Even with this schedule, lifestyle is generally considered to be a benefit of this specialty: "I work hard when I'm on and am uninterrupted when I'm off."

What Abilities and Talents Are Important in Anesthesiology?

The anesthesiologist's ability to pay attention to details for long periods of time is of paramount importance, according to respondents. "It is crucial that an anesthesiologist be able to concentrate and direct his or her attention on the patient at all times during an operation."

Accuracy and precision involving careful preparation and in-depth assessment of problems are essential—"One needs the ability to collect data and act decisively, to process information so as to see the big picture, to use scientific principles to bring order out of chaos, and to relate basic science information to clinical situations." Also, one must be able to react to rapidly changing clinical situations and to work efficiently with a great variety of personalities. Manual dexterity is imperative in order to perform procedures. Contact with individual patients may be short so it is an asset to have the ability to develop rapport quickly.

For those anesthesiologists choosing to become pain management specialists, counseling skills are imperative.

What Personality Traits Best Characterize Anesthesiologists?

Anesthesiologists describe themselves as patient and able to organize their thoughts and actions. Long hours in the operating room can be very stressful unless the anesthesiologist approaches each situation as a specific challenge. One respondent describes his colleagues as "easy going individuals who can tolerate a great deal of noxious and perplexing stimuli in the environment and still be able to carry out their functions." Another says that anesthesiologists are "team players who do not need external accolades in recognition of their work; who derive their satisfaction from their own observations of the results of their work." Ideally, the anesthesiologist should be "assertive with strong ego formation." One respondent says, "It may not be essential, but it is surely useful to be a cheerful person."

What Advice Would You Give a Medical Student Interested in Anesthesiology?

In addition to a "broad medical background," you are advised to "take an elective of at least one month's duration during the third or fourth year of medical school. Spend as much time as possible with one anesthesiologist, and not just in the operating room." Also, take electives in cardiology and pulmonary medicine to complement a necessary interest in physiology and pharmacology.

A residency director observes that some individuals choose anesthesiology with the misconception that it provides an "easier life." He thinks this is a mistaken concept and the wrong reason to choose a specialty.

In summary, "If one enjoys evaluating patients, appreciating and recognizing physiologic changes, is particularly interested in cardiopulmonary physiology and pharmacology, can make decisions and take actions quickly, and has sufficient ego function to tolerate a lack of appropriate regard for one's talents, he or she may be able to become a good anesthesiologist."

What Are the Future Challenges to Anesthesiology?

Respondents' answers reflect their types of practices: "Safe provision of pain relief for women in labor with even fewer side effects than currently is the case" (from an obstetrical anesthesiologist); "a wide range of research areas . . . particularly as the specialty interfaces with other disciplines such as surgery, bioengineering, medicine, and even veterinary science" (from an academician); "to administer *every* anesthetic and eliminate the use of nurse anesthetists" (from a private practitioner). Another anesthesiologist advocates MD/CRNA team care as a model to be offered in residency "because that's the way private practice anesthesiology is practiced in most parts of the country."

Other challenges include "avoiding adverse effects from meddlesome governmental regulations"; "acute care of patients outside the operating room"; "the management of chronic pain"; "greater understanding of normal physiological response to medication and stress"; "the use of computers, calculators, and advanced electronic monitoring equipment in the routine care of the anesthetized patient"; and "improved techniques of administering anesthesia: better intravenous techniques, more cost effective approach to general anesthesia, better ability to determine level of anesthesia and amounts of inhalation agent being administered to patients."

A report of a recent survey [3] reports that anesthesiologists (particularly residents) had high burnout scores. This is attributed to "increasing production pressure and staff shortages, care of extremely ill patients, and work with extreme responsibility."

REFERENCES

1. Coombs RH. *Mastering medicine.* New York: The Free Press. 1978, p. 207.
2. www.merritthawkins.com/pdf/2005_ModernHealthcare_ PhysicianCompensation_Review.pdf; accessed December 26, 2010.
3. Hyman SA, Michaels DR, Berry JM, et al. Risk of burnout in perioperative physicians. Anesthesiology 2011; 114(1):194-204.

Job Values Selection of Anesthesiologists

You can complete the questionnaires and obtain your scores for all specialties online at http://www.sdn.net, or compare your job values (as recorded in the Appendix) with the job values of anesthesiologist respondents on the next page.

Anesthesiologists' Choices:	My Choices:
1. Taking care of people	1. _____
2. Decision making	2. _____
3. Working with my mind	3. _____
4. Working with my hands	4. _____

No one chose: Creativity, security, prestige, feedback from others

Summary Profile of Anesthesiologists (derived from questionnaire answers)	My Personal Profile as an Anesthesiologist				
They tend to:	I tend to: (circle one number)				
	Never	Rarely	Sometimes	Frequently	Always
Enjoy taking care of people	1	2	3	4	5
Have manual dexterity	1	2	3	4	5
Be team players	1	2	3	4	5
Have a long attention span	1	2	3	4	5
Need to see tangible results of their efforts quickly	1	2	3	4	5
Prefer a planned schedule	1	2	3	4	5
Value time off	1	2	3	4	5
Be easy going	1	2	3	4	5
Pay attention to details	1	2	3	4	5
Rely on experience rather than theory	1	2	3	4	5

Add total of numbers circled to get your TOTAL SCORE:_____

Transfer score to the Appendix.

Anesthesia

sounds like me_____

could be a possibility _____

doesn't sound like me at all _____

Colon and Rectal Surgery

FAST FACTS:

Number of positions matched in 2010 to start in 2011 : 79

Competiveness: Medium (78 % of US Applicants matched)

Length of training: 1- 2 years after successful completion of a five year general surgery residency program

Number of residency programs: 49

Number of residents in training: 73

Number in US Board Certified in Colon and Rectal Surgery: 249

Median compensation for all physicians in specialty: $277,441

Average work hours per week: 62

THIS SPECIALTY WAS CALLED PROCTOLOGY (DERIVED FROM the Greek word *proktos*, meaning anus) until 1961 when the name was changed to colon and rectal surgery to reflect a broader scope of interest. Recognized specialists in this field are defined by the American Board of Colon and Rectal Surgery as surgeons who ". . . have demonstrated detailed knowledge and skill in surgery of the intestinal tract, rectum, anal canal, and perianal area. They are able to deal surgically with contiguous organs and tissues secondarily involved by primary intestinal disease. Their training and experience have resulted in the development of special skills in the performance of endoscopic procedures of the rectum and colon."

Interest in and knowledge of this surgical subspecialty is rare among medical students. There are only a small number of academic training programs so there is little student exposure to physicians in this field until surgical residency training years.

Residency Information. Colon and rectal surgery has one of the longest training programs in medicine (equal in length to plastic and thoracic surgery). A first postgraduate year—usually in general surgery—is followed by four years of general surgery and a one- or two-year fellowship in colon and rectal surgery.

Board Certification. Certification by the American Board of Surgery is a prerequisite to examination by the American Board of Colon and Rectal Surgery.

Supply and Projections. The American Society of Colon and Rectal Surgeons gives encouragement to those considering this specialty, "The small number of training programs led to the education of a relatively few specialists in this field and while the number of programs has increased, it has not yet reached a level of producing enough colon and rectal surgeons to meet the growing patient demand."[1] A recent study[2] of Census projections on the aging of the US population combined with anticipated growth in colorectal surgical services raises concern about the supply of physicians trained in this specialty.

Economic Status and Types of Practice. The colon and rectal surgeons' income data are included under the category of "surgeons." Colon and rectal surgeons generally have high office expenses and high professional liability premiums.

Most colon and rectal surgeons are in private practice. The great majority of residencies are in private institutions rather than academic centers, resulting in few full-time academicians in this specialty.

Further Information. The American Society of Colon and Rectal Surgeons, 85 W. Algonquin Road, Suite 550, Arlington Heights, IL 60005. Telephone: 847-290-9184. Internet address: www.fascrs.org.

A COMPOSITE PICTURE OF THE COLON AND RECTAL SURGEON

Why Choose Colon and Rectal Surgery?

All respondents chose this specialty after medical school and were influenced by mentors in the field: "I was dead tired one night on call on the thoracic surgical service, which I thought I was interested in, when along came the happiest colorectal surgeon I ever saw. I realized that with surgery he was *curing* patients, not just palliating them, and they were and are the most appreciative patients around." Another says, "One of my surgical professors had an interest in colon and rectal surgery and he had suggested to me while we were discussing a patient with a rectal problem that I might consider looking into specializing in this field."

The respondents considered other surgical specialties but they found the other fields "overcrowded" (urology, ophthalmology, and general surgery) or "too depressing" (neurosurgery and thoracic surgery). Colon and rectal surgeons report that they would not want to practice specialties that involved primarily office practice or "long-standing problems that cannot be cured."

What Do You Like Most About Colon and Rectal Surgery?

"The chance to offer a surgical cure for significant disabling problems." All respondents specifically enjoy surgery and the resulting "satisfaction of being able to help patients."

In addition, colon and rectal surgeons enjoy being tertiary consultants—"being well trained in a specific field" and "helping people with problems unsolved by others."

What Do You Like Least About Colon and Rectal Surgery?

Similar answers as those of the general surgeons were recorded: paperwork, long hours, and dealing with terminal problems. As a subspecialist, one respondent does not enjoy doing general surgery as part of his office association responsibility.

What Is Your Typical Daily Schedule?

Like other surgeons, colon and rectal surgeons have a long working day, starting as early as 6:30 AM and continuing until evening. Their patient population includes all age groups, but the majority of patients are middle-age to elderly. There is generally a mix of 60 percent ano-rectal problems and 40 percent colon problems. "On call" varies with the type of practice arrangement: One respondent is responsible for after-hours calls every other night and every other weekend; another is "always on call for colon or rectal problems through the emergency room, but I do not have to see much there since most are sent to my office for a regular visit"; and another has call one weekend in five with second call for emergency surgery every third weekend. Overall, they report "very few night calls in this specialty."

What Abilities and Talents Are Important in Colon and Rectal Surgery?

All respondents said "manual dexterity" was important. In addition, the abilities and talents are the same as those of a general surgeon.

What Personality Traits Best Characterize Colon and Rectal Surgeons?

Respondents report themselves as decisive, "calm but firm," and, unlike the surgical stereotype, "easy-going."

What Advice Would You Give a Medical Student Interested in Colon and Rectal Surgery?

You are advised to wait until later in your career to make a firm decision about this subspecialty field. "You first must decide on general surgery as a residency and it will expose you to colon and rectal problems as well as endoscopy."

There is encouragement to prospective specialists in this field as it is characterized as "a good uncrowded specialty."

What Are the Future Challenges to Colon and Rectal Surgery?

Two areas stand out: (1) the need to produce more specialists in the field by increasing the number of residency positions, and (2) the advancements in the diagnosis of and treatment of colon cancer and inflammatory bowel disease.

REFERENCES

1. *Colon and rectal surgery.* Booklet published annually by the American Society of Colon and Rectal Surgeons, Arlington Heights, IL.
2. Etzioni DA, Beart RW Jr., Madoff RD, Ault GT. Impact of the aging population on the demand for colorectal procedures. *Dis Colon Rectum;* 2009 Apr; 52(4):583-590.

Job Values Selection of Colon and Rectal Surgeons

You can complete the questionnaires and obtain your scores for all specialties online at http://www.sdn.net, or compare your job values (as recorded in the Appendix) with the job values of colon and rectal surgeon respondents below:

Colon and Rectal Surgeons' Choices:	My Choices:
1. Working with my hands	1. _____
2. Working with people	2. _____
3. Independence	3. _____
4. Taking care of people	4. _____

None of the respondents chose: Variety, decision making, prestige, good income, sufficient time off, or feedback from others

Summary Profile of Colon and Rectal Surgeons (derived from questionnaire answers)	My Personal Profile as a Colon and Rectal Surgeon

They tend to:	I tend to: (circle one number)				
	Never	Rarely	Sometimes	Frequently	Always
Be energized by people	1	2	3	4	5
Value independence highly	1	2	3	4	5
Have manual dexterity	1	2	3	4	5
Act decisively	1	2	3	4	5
Need to see tangible results of their efforts quickly	1	2	3	4	5
Be easy going	1	2	3	4	5
Enjoy caring for people	1	2	3	4	5
Prefer a planned schedule	1	2	3	4	5
Enjoy being an "expert"	1	2	3	4	5
Be comfortable doing the same activity repeatedly	1	2	3	4	5

Add total of numbers circled to get your TOTAL SCORE: _____

Transfer score to the Appendix.

Colon and rectal surgery

    sounds like me _____

    could be a possibility _____

    doesn't sound like me at all _____

Dermatology

FAST FACTS:

Number of first year positions offered in the NRMP in 2011 : 28

2011 US grads fill rate for first year positions in the NRMP: 92.9%

Number of second year positions offered in the NRMP in 2011 : 334

2011 US grads fill rate for second year positions in the NRMP: 82.3%

Length of training: 4 years, including a broad-based PGY-1 year of training

Number of residency programs: 12 have first year entry positions; 107 have second year entry positions

Number of residents in training: 883

Competitiveness: Highest

Competitive applicants have: membership in AOA; research, including published articles; interest in academics

US senior matched applicants' mean USMLE Step 1 score: 242

US senior matched applicants' mean USMLE Step 2 CK score: 251

Number in US Board Certified in Dermatology: 8,340

Starting median compensation in clinical practice: $237,500

Median compensation for mid-to late career in specialty: $350,000

Average work hours per week: 45

DERMATOLOGY DEALS WITH THE MEDICAL ASPECTS (AND sometimes surgical treatment) of skin disorders and diseases. In addition, dermatologists provide valuable medical therapy and emotional support for many individuals with chronic skin diseases. Some physicians view their colleagues in dermatology as having an "easier" life. This view is held even among some medical students who, in Coombs' study, describe dermatologists as "'medical cop-outs'—practitioners who are neither dedicated nor clinically involved in primary patient care."[1]

However, medical students usually have little contact with dermatologists and this harsh indictment is balanced by those primary care and subspecialty physicians who rely on the dermatologist's diagnostic skills. Dermatologists are playing a greater role in research as they become involved in all areas of the basic sciences.

Residency Information. You interview at the end of your fourth year for a position starting at the end of your internship year. The training in dermatology is three years, plus a first year of broad-based clinical training. The first year may be taken in a number of disciplines, including internal medicine, surgery, family medicine, and pediatrics. There are a small number of American Osteopathic Association (AOA) approved residency programs. Residency directors consider applicants highly who are AOA members, have high Board scores and grades and have research interests including published articles.

After completing either a dermatology or pathology residency, advanced training may be taken in a one- or two-year dermatopathology fellowship program. About 60 positions are offered annually.

Board Certification. After successfully completing four years of post-graduate training, including three years of dermatology, you may apply to take the certifying examination. The examination consists of two parts, one is written and the other uses visual aids and microscopic sections to assess knowledge.

A special qualification in dermatopathology is awarded jointly by the American Board of Dermatology and the American Board of Pathology. Basic certification by one of these two boards plus an additional one or two years of training in dermatopathology or basic certification by *both* boards are the prerequisites for application for certification.

The American Board of Dermatology also offers a special quali-fication in dermatopathology, pediatric dermatology and clinical and laboratory dermatological immunology.

Supply and Projections. Supply currently only slightly exceeds demand.[2] However, people today want cosmetic procedures and are more aware of skin cancers, creating consumer demand for dermatologists.

Economic Status and Types of Practice. The income of derma-tologists varies according to the practice setting and the types of ac-tivities. Dermatologists who are more procedure oriented will earn more money than those who focus on the diagnostic and psychological aspects of their patients' symptoms.

Dermatology is primarily an office-based specialty and most phy-sicians in this field are in private practice. Since there is infrequent need for after-hours coverage, many dermatologists are in solo practice. There are also opportunities in research and industry.

Further Information. The American Academy of Dermatology, P.O. Box 4014, Schaumburg, IL 60168. Telephone: (847) 330-0230. Internet address: www.aad.org.

A section of the Academy's web site offers information about programs and a "core curriculum" for medical students. There is a mentoring program for minority student members.

A COMPOSITE PICTURE OF THE DERMATOLOGIST
Why Choose Dermatology?

The diversity of the work and favorable working conditions were strong attractions for all respondents: "The most appealing aspect of dermatology . . . is the wide variety of skin disorders in all types of patient populations"; "The hours, lack of night call, dealing with both sexes, all age groups, and with a diversity of diagnoses and treatment methods were all appealing."

Respondents report that they do not enjoy "high pressure/emergency work or specialties that involve seriously ill patients." Allergy and im-munology, to one respondent, covers similar areas of medicine, but is "too restrictive."

What Do You Like Most About Dermatology?

The ability to help patients in most instances and the almost immediate positive feedback because "results are visible to both me and the patient" are enjoyable aspects of dermatology. Other positive reasons include "the lack of call at home," "correlating clinical findings with pathology," and "the challenge of seeing patients with a variety of problems—pediatric, geriatric, psychiatric, surgical, and immunologic disorders are all part of the daily fare of dermatology." The majority of dermatologists (56.1 percent) report themselves as "very satisfied" with only 10.8 percent "dissatisfied." [3]

What Do You Like Least About Dermatology?

No one could think of anything they didn't like about the activities involved in dermatology. Some respondents believed that there is a lack of respect for their specialty by other colleagues.

What Is Your Typical Daily Schedule?

Dermatologists spend most or all of their typical eight-hour day in the office. They may be called to the hospital for a consultation, but it is rare for them to have their own hospitalized patients. After-hour calls are rare and most can be handled over the telephone. The patient population is described as "intelligent and highly motivated." The most common problems are acne, psoriasis, and eczematous dermatitis. Surgical procedures are a significant part of the practice of dermatology.

What Abilities and Talents Are Important in Dermatology?

Keen observational and listening skills need to be developed. "It is important to be able to accurately see and feel the disorder and also be aware of the patient's perceptions of the disease." Manual dexterity is needed to perform surgical procedures, but one respondent says, "My lack of dexterity in excisional surgery and suturing led me into cryosurgery and has made dermatology far more interesting for me than if I had the ability to excise and suture well."

What Personality Traits Best Characterize Dermatologists?

This specialty seems to attract a diversity of personality types. Some respondents describe themselves as "intellectually motivated"; others see themselves as more psychologically oriented, easily able to empathize with patients. The Myers-Briggs Type Indicator data[4] report this duality of personality types in dermatology: "This specialty may attract physicians with two quite different types of interests—a practical and matter-of-fact group who are likely to stress the highly differentiated recognition of lesions and rashes . . . and a psychologically minded group who are more likely to approach treatment through the emotions, such as by ventilating hostility."

What Advice Would You Give a Medical Student Interested in Dermatology?

"Plan early and have an outstanding record since residency positions are at a premium." Since dermatology is not a required elective in the medical school curriculum, you are advised to get some experience by taking electives in teaching clinics, spending time with a community dermatologist, or doing research.

What Are the Future Challenges to Dermatology?

The greater emphasis on research and surgery will change dermatology from "a strictly medical specialty" in the years to come, according to one respondent. Concerns are raised about "turf battles" with other specialties and "the proliferation of new types of health insurance that limit direct access to dermatologists by patients since they will have to be referred by primary care physicians." Ackerman[5] issues a warning about the diminishing appeal of practicing dermatopathology citing the "surge to dermatologic surgery which is more lucrative."

REFERENCES

1. Coombs RH. *Mastering medicine.* New York: The Free Press, 1978, p. 206.

2. Resneck J. Too few or too many dermatologists?: difficulties in anticipating optimal workforce size. Arch Dermatol 2001; 137:1295-1301.
3. Leigh JP, Kravitz RL, Schembri M, Samuels SJ,, Mobley S. Physician career satisfaction across specialties. *Arch Intern Med* 2002; 162:1577-1584.
4. McCaulley MH. The Myers longitudinal medical study. Mono–graph I. Gainesville, FL: 1978, pp. 234–235.
5. Ackerman AB. Dermatology awake—dermatopathology is in peril. *J Am Acad Dermatol* 1991;25(1):128–130.

Job Values Selection of Dermatologists

You can complete the questionnaires and obtain your scores for all specialties online at http://www.sdn.net, or compare your job values (as recorded in the Appendix) with the job values of dermatologist respondents below:

Dermatologists' Choices:	My Choices:
1. Independence	1. _____
2. Variety	2. _____
3. Working with people	3. _____
4. Sufficient time off	4. _____

No one chose: Prestige

Summary Profile of Dermatologists (derived from questionnaire answers)	My Personal Profile as a Dermatologist				
They tend to:	I tend to: (circle one number)				
	Never	Rarely	Sometimes	Frequently	Always
Value time off	1	2	3	4	5
Prefer a planned schedule	1	2	3	4	5
Have interests outside of medicine	1	2	3	4	5
Be easy going	1	2	3	4	5
Value independence highly	1	2	3	4	5
Have good observational skills	1	2	3	4	5
Be interested in people	1	2	3	4	5
Have good listening skills/ interested in listening	1	2	3	4	5
Like complex problem solving	1	2	3	4	5
Need to see tangible results of their efforts quickly	1	2	3	4	5

Add total of numbers circled to get your TOTAL SCORE:_____

Transfer score to the Appendix.

Dermatology

sounds like me_____

could be a possibility_____

doesn't sound like me at all_____

Emergency Medicine

Number of first year positions offered in the NRMP in 2011: 1,607

2011 US grad fill rate for the first year positions in the NRMP: 78.9%

Number of second year positions offered in the NRMP in 2011: 19

2011 US grad fill rate for the second year positions in the NRMP: 47.4%

Length of training: years: 3 BUT there are also 3 year programs that begin in PGY-2 and 4 year categorical programs.

Number of residency programs: 150 offered first year entry positions; 3 offered second year entry positions

Number of residents in training: 3,676

Competitiveness: Very high

Competitive applicants have: high grades, experience in a clinical emergency department, letters of recommendation from emergency medicine faculty, good interview skills

US senior matched applicants' mean USMLE Step 1 score is: 222

US senior matched applicants' mean USMLE Step 2 CK score: 230

Number in US Board Certified in Emergency Medicine: 17,787

Range of compensation: $188,000- $246,000 (depends upon amount of work done)

Average work hours per week: 45

"The new kid on the block." "The fastest growing medical specialty." "The opportunity to be a 'real doctor.' " These are statements often used to describe the specialty of emergency medicine, one of the most popular residency choices among the top-ranked graduates of medical schools.

Emergency medicine's emphasis is on prehospital care and the acute care aspects of the other specialties. One emergency medicine physician says, "Its uniqueness lies in style rather than substance."[1] The emergency medicine physician is defined by the American College of Emergency Physicians (ACEM) as "one who is a specialist in breadth, whose training is focused on the acute and the life-threatening aspects of medical care, and who, by nature of his practice, is available when the patient needs him." The American Medical Association (AMA) House of Delegates defines the emergency medicine physician as the one who recognizes, evaluates, and cares for patients who are acutely ill or injured; administers, researches, and teaches emergency medical care; directs patients to follow-up care in or out of the hospital; provides emergency care, when requested, to hospitalized patients; and manages the emergency medical system for prehospital emergency care. "In a practical sense, the emergency physician functions both as the manager of the emergency department and as the clinician most apt to first see the injured patient."[2]

Residency Information. In the past 10 years the number of residency positions offered has risen sharply and the number of US seniors matching in this specialty has risen 60.5%. [3] The majority of emergency medicine programs begin in the first year. Those programs beginning in the second year require a transitional, internal medicine, family medicine, or surgery internship year and you apply through the NRMP in the fall of your internship. Training in emergency medicine has opportunities for additional training available in critical care, toxicology, administration, and research. A pediatric emergency medicine fellowship is obtained through the NRMP Specialties Matching Service. There are five-year combined residencies in emergency medicine-family medicine, emergency medicine-internal medicine and emergency medicine-pediatrics.

Osteopathic residency positions are available in 43 American Osteopathic Association-approved programs.

Board Certification. You must complete at least three years of emergency medicine residency training to be eligible for board certification. There are double-boarded physicians in emergency medicine because prior to 1988 you could qualify for certification based on practice experience, and many who entered this specialty had already obtained board certification in another area of medicine.

Subspecialty certifications in emergency medical services (approved in December 2010), hospice and palliative care, medical toxicology, pediatric emergency medicine, sports medicine, and undersea and hyperbaric medicine are offered.

Supply and Projections. AMA data may not reflect fully the number of physicians working in emergency medicine settings. The AMA data report that 31,722 physicians self-identify themselves as emergency medicine physicians; however, twelve years ago a comprehensive survey of 942 hospitals[4] reported that there were approximately 32,000 physicians working in emergency departments in the United States. In that study, 83 percent were men, and the average age was 42 years. Forty-six percent were certified by the American Board of Emergency Medicine (ABEM); 42 percent were trained or certified in other medical specialties. Of the nonemergency medicine–trained physicians working in the specialty, the largest number was trained in family medicine (32 percent) and internal medicine (28 percent). Presumably, there are even more emergency physicians because the survey did not include clinicians who were employed elsewhere, such as in occupational settings, cruise ships, and free-standing urgent care centers. It also did not include those in administrative, teaching, or government positions.

Projections indicate a shortage of emergency medicine physicians for at least several decades because the annual number of physicians leaving the field for administrative or nonmedical careers or retirement will soon equal the number of resident graduates each year.[5]

Economic Status and Types of Practice. Good income has been associated with emergency medicine since the advent of two factors: fee-for-service and third-party reimbursement as payment for emergency room services. An emergency medicine physician may be a salaried employee of a hospital, a member of a group of physicians providing emergency medicine coverage on a fee-for-service basis to one or more hospitals, or under contract to a national group which provides emergency room coverage for a hospital. Earnings are related to number of hours worked and number of patients seen and may vary according to location.

Further Information. The American College of Emergency Physicians, 1125 Executive Circle, Irving, TX 75038. Telephone: (800) 798-1822. Internet address: www.acep.org. Students can join ACEP through their affiliated resident association, the Emergency Medicine Medical Resident Association.

The American College of Osteopathic Emergency Physicians, 142 E. Ontario Street, Suite 218, Chicago, IL 60611-2818. Telephone: (312) 587-3709. There is a link for DO students that offers opportunities to attend national conferences and a mentorship program.

A COMPOSITE PICTURE OF THE EMERGENCY MEDICINE PHYSICIAN

Why Choose Emergency Medicine?

A diverse group calls themselves emergency medicine physicians: residents moonlighting, recent residency graduates exploring their options prior to opening a private practice, older physicians wishing to wind down their professional careers. However, there is a growing nucleus of physicians who are committed to this specialty as a career. Among these, many are making their specialty decision during, or even before, medical school and they have been found to be "relatively uninfluenced by professors, fellow students, or peers." Instead, it is their *experience* as they rotate through the emergency service that is a major influence. Also, many medical students ". . . choose emergency medicine precisely because of the amount of control one has over one's practice. The freedom to be mobile, to choose your hours, and not be bound to the business of setting up a practice, lends itself to a quality lifestyle."[6]

The primary care specialties of family medicine, general internal medicine, and pediatrics are characterized as "not exciting enough," "too much office practice routine," and "too many demands on my personal life." Also, respondents would not want to practice pathology and radiology—"no patient contact"; neurology—"too esoteric, cerebral, non-action oriented"; or nephrology or oncology—"mostly inpatient medical chronic disease." Some had considered surgery, but were turned off by the long years of training, the frequent night calls, and ". . . the amount of routine work which I found boring." Orthopaedics is "too narrow a field" and obstetrics and gynecology "only treats women."

What Do You Like Most About Emergency Medicine?

The appeal of emergency medicine is in both the nature of the work—the fast pace, the unpredictability, the variety of people and problems—and the regular hours—"I work hard when I'm on and am completely off when I'm not working." Emergency medicine physicians reports themselves to be slightly more satisfied than all physicians with 44.4% "very satisfied" and 13.3% "dissatisfied." [7]

What Do You Like Least About Emergency Medicine?

A high burnout rate has been attributed to built-in stresses: shift work involves the necessity of night as well as day work patterns, there is little positive feedback from patients and no continuity of care, and patients may even be abusive. Also, the physician sometimes must quickly manage unfamiliar situations.

However, until recently, physicians often have come into emergency medicine with the intention of staying only a short time and so longevity has been brief. Emergency medicine was seen as an "escape" from other areas of medicine rather than the positive choice it has become for many today.

What Is Your Typical Daily Schedule?

There are many different types of work schedules, but a frequently described one is the 12-hour shift, three to four times a week. A physician may be on duty for two weeks of days (7:00 AM to 7:00 PM) and two weeks of nights (7:00 PM to 7:00 AM.) For some, there are no on-call duties; for others, there is back-up call in case the emergency room becomes unusually busy.

There are no typical daily problems. "I may see one true emergency after another or all chronic patients with colds, sore throats, etc." The population served is a cross-section of the general populace, "similar to those seen in family medicine."

Many emergency medicine physicians are involved in community activities related to emergency medical care. They help in training emergency medical technicians, direct ambulance services, teach cardiopulmonary resuscitation courses, and participate in continuing medical education courses for health professionals.

What Abilities and Talents Are Important in Emergency Medicine?

This specialty requires certain training and interests not found in all physicians. An emergency medicine physician needs a "sound base of medical knowledge and skills in manipulative areas, particularly as applies to IV access, airway management, surgical techniques, and minor orthopedics techniques."

This is a team-oriented specialty and the physician needs to have strong leadership abilities as well as "diplomacy in dealing with other physicians and nurses."

What Personality Traits Best Characterize Emergency Medicine Physicians?

A sample of 157 ACEP members who took the Myers-Briggs Type Indicator showed a significant overrepresentation of individuals who are "action-oriented, quick to determine the possibilities inherent in the situation, coolly logical under stressful circumstances, and well suited to dealing with the unexpected as emergencies arise."[7]

"The best practitioners are cool, calm, and collected." "One must be able to organize multiple things simultaneously—to handle stress, a variety of decisions and problems at once." "Decisiveness, often without complete information and compassion for many types of people" are valued traits. To have "a sense of humor" helps.

One emergency medicine physician describes himself as having "an interest in active procedures, rather than in prolonged diagnostic procedures and modes."

What Advice Would You Give a Medical Student Interested in Emergency Medicine?

"Be prepared for heavy competition for choice positions in residency training and practice." As the newest specialty, emergency medicine is attracting medical student interest, but the advice is cautionary. "Take a hard look at your career goals and what you want out of your profession. Some physicians don't feel complete if they don't have their *own* patients."

Medical students are advised to "take a clinical elective in emergency medicine at a site where there is a residency program," "develop a good fund of knowledge and of manipulative skills—there isn't a lot of time to look things up or start training when a true emergency presents itself," and "spend holidays and weekends in an emergency department."

What Are the Future Challenges to Emergency Medicine?

Respondents see challenges in the improvement of prehospital care through involvement with emergency medical systems; the advent of new technologies; and the creation of subspecialties within emergency medicine such as disaster medicine, toxicology, and trauma. Many agree that clinical research is needed in this field, as well as studies on how to contain costs and improve health care delivery.

Residency programs are concentrated in a small number of states, and data indicate that 50 percent of the graduates remain in the city where they train.[8] The challenge is to improve the geographic distribution to meet the needs of the nation as emergency medicine has become the "safety net" for health care.

REFERENCES

1. Leitzell JD. Sounding boards: An uncertain future. *N Engl J Med* 1981;304:477–480.
2. Thompson CT. The emergency physician, the trauma surgeon, and the trauma center. *Ann Emer Med* 1983;12:235–237.
3. Salsberg E. National Physician Workforce Trends. Presentation at the American College of Emergency Physicians, Washington, DC, April 22, 2008.
4. Moorhead JC, Gallery ME, Mannle T et al. A study of the workforce in emergency medicine. *Ann Emer Med* 1998;31(5):595–607.
5. Holliman CJ, Wuerz RC, Hirshberg AJ. Analysis of factors affecting U.S. emergency physician workforce projections. *Acad Emer Med* 1997;4(7):731–735.
6. Hallagan L. Rites of passage. *Life in Medicine* 1996;3(5):23.
7. Leigh JP, Kravitz RL, Schembri M, Samuels SJ,, Mobley S. Physician career satisfaction across specialties. *Arch Intern Med* 2002; 162:1577-1584.
8. Henderson RS, Harris DL. Psychological types of emergency physicians as measured by the MBTI. *J Psyc Type* 1991;21:59–61.
9. Steele MT, Schwab RA, McNamara RM et al. Emergency medicine resident choice of practice location. *Ann Emer Med* 1998;31:351–357.

Job Values Selection of Emergency Medicine Physicians

You can complete the questionnaires and obtain your scores for all specialties online at http://www.sdn.net, or compare your job values (as recorded in the Appendix) with the job values of emergency medicine respondents below:

Emergency Medicine Physicians' Choices:	My Choices:
1. Variety	1. _____
2. Sufficient time off	2. _____
3. Good income	3. _____
3. Independence	4. _____
(there is a tie for third place)	

No one chose: Creativity, security, prestige, achievement, working with my hands, feedback from others

Summary Profile of Emergency Medicine Physicians (derived from questionnaire answers)	My Personal Profile as an Emergency Medicine Physician				
They tend to:	**I tend to: (circle one number)**				
	Never	Rarely	Sometimes	Frequently	Always
Become bored with repetitive activity	1	2	3	4	5
Value time off	1	2	3	4	5
Act decisively	1	2	3	4	5
Have interests outside of medicine	1	2	3	4	5
Rely on experience rather than theory	1	2	3	4	5
Be adventurous/like challenges	1	2	3	4	5
Communicate well	1	2	3	4	5
Be a leader	1	2	3	4	5
Want quick results	1	2	3	4	5
Be able to do more than one thing at a time	1	2	3	4	5

Add total of numbers circled to get your TOTAL SCORE: _____

Transfer score to the Appendix.

Emergency medicine

sounds like me _____

could be a possibility _____

doesn't sound like me at all _____

Family Medicine

FAST FACTS:

Number of first year positions offered in the NRMP in 2011: 2,708
2011 US grad fill rate in the NRMP: 48 %
Length of training: 3 years
Number of residency programs: 453
Number of residents in training: 9,799
Competitiveness: low to moderate, depending upon location
Competitive applicants have: good interpersonal skills in the residency interview, evidence of community service
US senior matched applicants' mean Step 1 score: 214
US senior matched applicants' mean step 2 score: 223
Number in US Board Certified in Family Medicine: 60,298
Range of compensation: $150,000 – $177,000; Average - $175,000; if offering maternity care - $200,000
Average work hours per week: 52

FOR MANY PEOPLE THE IMAGE OF THE PHYSICIAN IS THAT of the old-time country doctor. Prior to World War II, the great majority of physicians were general practitioners located in both rural and urban settings who incorporated medicine, surgery, obstetrics, and psychiatry into their practices. Medical students often start their training believing that they would like to be family physicians or "generalists."

Formerly called "family practice," family medicine was recognized in 1969 as the twentieth medical specialty and residencies were developed in response to public need for well-trained generalist physicians. The official definition is: "family medicine is the medical specialty which provides continuing, comprehensive health care for the individual and family. It is a specialty in breadth that integrates the biological, clinical and behavioral sciences. The scope of family medicine encompasses all ages, both sexes, each organ system and every disease entity."

Today's family physician is trained to provide primary health care, coordinate the care of all family members with other specialized physicians and community services, teach preventive medicine to patients, and be the patient's advocate in all aspects of health care delivery.[1] Primarily, the family physician differs from the "general practice" physician not only in formal residency training but also in the focus of delivering health care in the context of family rather than the patient alone.

Residency Information. The three years of residency training combine experience in both the hospital and ambulatory care settings. However, much time is spent in a family medicine center, which is intended to mirror a private practice setting. The curriculum includes the study of adult medicine, surgery, child health, maternal and women's health, behavioral science, gerontology, community medicine, diagnostic imaging, and practice management. Continuity of family care is stressed and each resident has his or her own panel of patients for the three years of training.

There are residency programs in every state; most are in community hospitals rather than in medical school/university settings. In deciding whether to invite a student for an interview, the personal statement is a key factor. The interview is, however, is "most valuable" in ranking a student in the residency match since, as one residency director writes, "We value interpersonal skills very highly." Overall academic standing, especially on clinical clerkships, is a factor in getting an interview in the more competitive programs.

An increasing number of fellowship programs—in geriatrics, sports medicine, adolescent medicine, hospice and palliative care, integrative medicine, women's health, research, administration, and health policy—are being offered after completion of residency. Osteopathic fellowships are offered in geriatrics and manipulative medicine.

Board Certification. Upon successful completion of a three-year family medicine residency program, with the latter two years of training required to be completed in the same accredited program, you may apply to take the written certification examination. The American Board of Family Medicine was the first specialty board to require re-certification to maintain diplomate status.

Certificates of Added Qualification are offered after successful completion of fellowships in adolescent medicine, geriatric medicine, hospice and palliative care, sleep medicine and sports medicine. (See separate chapters on adolescent medicine, geriatrics, hospice and palliative medicine and sports medicine in Part 3 of this book.)

Supply and Projections. Thirty-nine percent of family physicians are women, but this number will soon increase because 56 percent of current family medicine residents are women. Today, virtually all physicians who choose family medicine as a specialty complete the three-year residency program, thereby eliminating what was formerly known as "general practice" for which a graduate of a medical school can be licensed, but not board-certified in any specialty. In the 33 years from 1975 to 2008 those who identified themselves as general practitioners declined in number by 77.4 percent.[2]

A workforce blueprint for 2020 indicates an increased need for family physicians due to the aging population, increasing part-time practice, and a serious undersupply in inner-city and rural sites.[3]

Economic Status and Types of Practice. The median income range for family physicians is $150,000–$177,000 with geographic variations and higher for those who do obstetrics. Although liability insurance costs are lower than for surgical specialties, those family physicians who include obstetrics as part of their practices have higher premiums than those who do not. Also, like pediatrics, a good deal of professional time involves counseling and patient education, services that are not generously reimbursed by third-party payers.

Only 12.8 percent of active members of AAFP have settled in communities smaller than 20,000, and 2 percent in towns of fewer than 2500. In contrast, 64.9 percent of all family physicians practice in cities with more than 250,000 population.[4] Health maintenance organizations (HMOs) are often interested in employing family physicians because it is believed that having a family physician as the entry into the health care system will be more efficient and cost-effective.[5] There are many career opportunities for family physicians—private practice, academics, school health, sports medicine, and international medicine to name a few.

Further Information. The American Academy of Family Physicians, 11400 Tomahawk Creek Parkway, Leawood, KS 66211. Telephone: (800) 274-2237. Internet address: www.aafp.org. Student membership is available for free. There is a student website www.fmig.net which gives information on Family Medicine Interest Group activities and residency application.

The American College of Osteopathic Family Physicians, 330 E. Algonquin Road, Suite 2, Arlington Heights, IL 60005. Telephone: (800) 323-0794. Internet address: www.acofp.org.

A COMPOSITE PICTURE OF THE FAMILY PHYSICIAN

Some respondents to the questionnaire graduated from medical school prior to the inception of family medicine residencies and started practice as general practitioners. However, all have identified themselves today as family physicians and are certified by the American Board of Family Medicine.

Why Choose Family Medicine?

Most respondents chose this specialty even before they started medical school. Some had their own family physicians as role models; others had formed an image of themselves working with people and providing broad-based medical care. Initial plans were often reinforced by clinical experiences: "A summer preceptorship with a general practitioner in Altoona, Pennsylvania, firmly convinced me that general practice was the way to go"; "my decision was finalized after a six-week preceptorship during the summer between my first and second years of medical school."

Specifically appealing is the variety of practice opportunities and experiences; other primary care specialties were rejected because they were judged to be too narrow in scope. "I considered pediatrics, but wished to have more than social contact with adults. I considered internal medicine, but I wanted a pediatric component to my practice." Pathology and radiology are considered to have too little contact with people, while psychiatry is seen as "too intense." Many respondents say that choosing another specialty would have meant giving up some area of medicine and they did not want to do that. Also there is a strong interest expressed in dealing with the entire family rather than one individual patient.

What Do You Like Most About Family Medicine?

The factors that were initially appealing about family medicine bring the greatest enjoyment. "Taking care of whole families—my practice is 50 percent pediatrics and this causes the young parents to come when they get sick and then often the grandparents will switch doctors so that the whole family can be cared for by the same physician." It is not only the patient care that they like, but also the relationships developed with patients and families: "the gratification of communicating closely with patients who generally trust and appreciate you and your treatment." Satisfaction levels are above the national average with 42.8 percent reporting "very satisfied" and 16.9 percent reporting "dissatisfied." [6]

What Do You Like Least About Family Medicine?

Ironically, some of the same aspects of family medicine that are most rewarding, both professionally and personally, can cause the most stress. Respondents report that close relationships with patients may cause emotional distress for the physician when a patient is dependent, demanding, or terminally ill. Even though respondents say that the numbers of "difficult patients" are small, they are a disturbing enough factor to include as a least-liked aspect of the specialty.

What Is Your Typical Daily Schedule?

Although family medicine is considered by many students to be a time-demanding specialty, the respondents report a working day of from 9 to 10 hours, fewer hours than most surgeons. What is disruptive for some family physicians, however, is their schedule during the day. A family physician may have to spend more time than scheduled with a patient or, if offering maternity care, leave an office full of patients to deliver a baby.

Some family physicians start and end their day with hospital rounds. Others, especially in large urban areas, only have an office-based practice. One respondent says, "Every day in the office is different. Some days are full of trauma and lacerations; some days, family planning and childbirth; some days, just a variety of problems." Family physicians manage over 90 percent of the problems in their offices. Even when a consultation is requested, the family physician will remain actively involved in the care of the patient, serving as the coordinator and advocate; and, ideally making "social visits" to their hospitalized patients.

In addition to office and hospital patient care, the family physician may be on staff at a nursing home, be medical director of a volunteer rescue squad, or serve as the local high school sports-team physician, involving after-office hours. On-call schedules vary according to the type of practice, and some respondents have found it more efficient to schedule evening and weekend office hours rather than deal with numerous telephone calls. Family physician respondents report a high level of participation on hospital and medical society committees and in volunteer service for their communities.

What Abilities and Talents Are Important in Family Medicine?

"The single most important talent, in my mind, is the ability to relate in a positive manner to people. . . ." This relationship includes not only patients, but also family members, consultants, and other health professionals.

The family physician is described as "an expert in the evaluation and management of common health problems . . ." [7] and, as such, needs to have wide, general knowledge and skills. Taylor [8] observes: "The physician who specializes in a limited area such as the eye or heart will approach medicine in the context of personal knowledge and experience; this physician will have personally encountered other cases of retinoblastoma or hyperaldosteronism. The family physician, on the other hand, approaches disease in the context of theory and application . . . the family doctor learns to approach clinical challenges in a problem-solving framework, working through solutions by applying basic principles of diagnosis and management."

Organizational skills to coordinate the practice, patients, and consultants; manual skills for procedures such as cast applications and minor surgery; and the ability to feel intellectually secure in the face of ambiguity are all valuable in family medicine.

What Personality Traits Best Characterize Family Physicians?

Respondents most often describe those in their specialty as "humanistic," "people-oriented," and "understanding." One respondent says, "gregarious or at least not introverted." In dealing with a large number of people each day it seems that it would be an advantage to communicate easily with people.

Family physicians also are characterized as "those who do not need to be the absolute expert in any area but rather like to be a 'front-line' physician." They see themselves as "conscientious and moderately compulsive."

What Advice Would You Give a Medical Student Interested in Family Medicine?

"I would advise a medical student to pursue a preceptorship in family medicine in a community practice setting. The true way to appreciate family medicine is to see it as it exists at the grass roots level." Students are advised to "make sure you can be content knowing 'a little about a lot' because it is virtually impossible to know all areas of medicine to the nth degree." Also, "obtain a good basic medical education . . . once in residency, maintain documentation of all training experiences."

What Are the Future Challenges to Family Medicine?

Many respondents express the need for family medicine to develop an academic research base and also to "maintain credibility in an era of exploding technology—it is important to keep up to date in the applications of technology and, at the same time, deal more effectively with the psychosocial needs of our patient population." "Outcomes data based on population medicine" is critically needed to demonstrate the quality of family medicine.

In practice settings, family physicians need to "develop competitive marketing skills without becoming cynical or rendering substandard medical care." There is concern expressed about maintaining hospital privileges in a time of increasing competition in medicine, and one respondent sees a challenge to family physicians "to assume a leadership role as the nature of primary health care delivery changes over the ensuing years."

REFERENCES

1. Taylor RB. Family practice: The specialty that puts it all together. *Med Student* 1984;11(1):8–13.
2. Physician Characteristics and Distribution in the US, 2010 Edition. American Medical Association. p. 441.
3. Bein B. AAFP's New Physician Workforce Report Repesents "Blueprint for Change." 10/2/2009. www.aafp.org, accessed January 15, 2011.
4. Facts About Family Medicine, Table 13. February 2010.American Academy of Family Physicians. www.aafp.org/online/en/home/aboutus/specialty/facts/13.printerview.html. accessed 12/22/10
5. Seifer SD, Troupin B, Rubenfeld G. Changes in marketplace demand for physicians. *JAMA* 1996;276(9):695-699.

6. Leigh JP, Kravitz RL, Schembri M, Samuels SJ,, Mobley S. Physician career satisfaction across specialties. *Arch Intern Med* 2002; 162:1577-1584.

7. McGaha AL, Garrett E, Jobe AC, Nalin P, et al. Responses to medical students' frequently asked questions about family medicine. *Am Fam Physician* 2007;76(1):99-106.

8. Taylor RB. What students ask about family practice. *Fam Med Teacher* 1980;12(5):20–21.

Job Values Selections of Family Physicians

You can complete the questionnaires and obtain your scores for all specialties online at http://www.sdn.net, or compare your job values (as recorded in the Appendix) with the job values of family physician respondents below:

Family Physicians' Choices:	My Choices:
1. Working with people	1. _____
2. Variety	2. _____
3. Creativity	3. _____
3. Independence	4. _____
(there is a tie for third place)	

No one chose: Prestige, working with my hands

Summary Profile of Family Physicians (derived from questionnaire answers)

My Personal Profile as a Family Physician

They tend to:

I tend to: (circle one number)

	Never	Rarely	Sometimes	Frequently	Always
Value independence highly	1	2	3	4	5
Communicate well	1	2	3	4	5
Be a leader	1	2	3	4	5
Want to do everything in medicine	1	2	3	4	5
Like to organize people	1	2	3	4	5
Like to coordinate care of patients and their families	1	2	3	4	5
Be content knowing "a little about a lot"	1	2	3	4	5
Enjoy being involved in their patients' lives	1	2	3	4	5
Tolerate the unknown	1	2	3	4	5
Accept schedule disruptions	1	2	3	4	5

Add total of numbers circled to get your TOTAL SCORE:_____

Transfer score to the Appendix.

Family medicine

sounds like me_____

could be a possibility_____

doesn't sound like me at all _____

Internal Medicine

THE NAMES OF MEDICAL SPECIALTIES REFER TO AREAS OF THE body (otolaryngology and dermatology), target population (pediatrics, family medicine, and the emerging areas of interest in adolescent medicine and geriatrics), techniques (surgery and radiology), and the setting of activities (occupational medicine and aerospace medicine). The specialty name of "internal medicine" does not fit into any of these categories and it has been a source of confusion to many. A survey of 552 first- and second-year medical students at three Michigan medical schools revealed that 31 percent did not have a well-defined image of the specialist in internal medicine.[1] They were unable to distinguish between an internist, a general practitioner, a family physician, and an intern, a situation that was cited by Coombs[2] two decades ago. Unfortunately, the confusion extended to knowledge about the kinds of medical care internists provide—with the majority of respondents (86 percent) identifying "old people" as the predominant patient population.

Concerns about the internist's image continue. In 1997 the American College of Physicians launched a three-year public education campaign to deliver the message to adults between the ages of 35 and 60 that internists are specially trained to take care of them. Goodman[3] advocates a change of name to "adult medicine."

Until the 1950s internists functioned as "consultants" to the larger number of general practitioners. The next two decades saw increasing subspecialization in internal medicine with an accompanying decline in the numbers of generalists providing primary care to patients. Training was primarily in treating hospitalized patients. Today that trend is being reversed because the Residency Review Committee for Internal Medicine requires at least 33 percent of training in the outpatient setting.

GENERAL INTERNAL MEDICINE

▮▮▮▮▮▮▮▮ FAST FACTS: ▮▮▮

Number of fellowship positions matched in 2010 to start in 2011: 79

Competitiveness: Medium (80% of US grads matched); helpful to have research experience or a residency at a large academic center

Length of training: 5 years (2 years after 3 years of internal medicine or pediatrics residency)

Number of fellowship programs: 79

Number of fellows in training: 219

Number in US Board Certified in Allergy and Immunology: 608

Number Board Certified in 2009: 145; Number Recertified in 2009: 203

Starting median compensation: $135,000

Median compensation for all physicians in specialty: $183,000

Mean # of hours weekly in patient care activities: 35.3

Mean # of hours weekly in professional activities: 40.7

I first will discuss the general internist—a physician who provides primary health care to adults full time and who is not trained in a subspecialty of internal medicine.

Residency Information. Training for the practice of general internal medicine is three years. You can choose a primary care (emphasis on ambulatory care and offering electives in women's health musculoskeletal issues or sports medicine or traditional (academic/hospital-based) track. Residents from either track can go into practice or do a subspecialty fellowship. Every year about 7000 first-year positions in internal medicine are offered through the National Resident Matching Program (NRMP); one third of these positions are for only one year (preliminary positions) to accommodate those planning to train in other specialties which match students starting in their second year of residency, such as anesthesiology and radiology.

The table below details the available combined residencies.

Combined Residencies	Number of Programs	Number of First Year Positions
Internal Medicine/Dermatology	8	6
Internal Medicine/ Emergency Medicine	12	24
Internal Medicine/Family Medicine	2	6
Internal Medicine/Medical Genetics	4	2
Internal Medicine/Neurology	6	2
Internal Medicine/Pediatrics	81	359
Internal Medicine/Preventive Medicine	8	7
Internal Medicine/Psychiatry	16	20

The most important factors in ranking applicants for one residency director are "global academic performance; performance during the medicine clerkship; and information about attitudes, behaviors, inter-personal skills; and outside activities."

Board Certification. After successful completion of three years of an internal medicine residency program, you may apply to take the written examination for board certification.

Supply and Projections. There are more board-certified internists than any other specialists in medicine, but this number includes sub-specialists as well as generalists in internal medicine. In practice, there are actually more physicians providing general internal medicine care to adult patients than any data show because about 36 percent of sub-specialists are spending an average of 27 percent of their time offering primary care services.[4]

Economic Status and Types of Practice. Salary offers to general internists are continuing to increase slightly and demand is steady. A wide variety of practice opportunities exist for a general internist. You may choose to practice alone or as part of a group, in an urban or rural setting, as a salaried employee or in a fee-for-service arrangement. Most general internists are involved in direct patient care in an office-based practice and are located in cities with populations of 25,000 or more. The largest group of combined residency graduates is in internal medicine/pediatrics (commonly called Med-Peds).

Further Information. The American College of Physicians, 190 N. Independence Mall West, Philadelphia, PA 19106-1572. Telephone: (800) 523-1546; (215) 351-2400. Internet address: www. acponline.org. A section of the website includes information about mentoring opportunities and residency selection. Student memberships are available.

The American College of Osteopathic Internists, 300 Fifth Street NE, Washington, DC 20002. Telephone: (202) 546-0095.

A COMPOSITE PICTURE OF THE GENERAL INTERNIST

Why Choose General Internal Medicine?

Physician respondents report selecting internal medicine while in medical school: "The internal medicine attendings and housestaff were excellent role models." Anwar[5] reports that internal medicine residents are influenced by both medical school professors and peers in making their career choice. Respondents say that the most appealing aspect of general internal medicine was "the variety of disease entities."

General internists report that they would not want to practice surgery: "I'm not action-oriented," "I'm a klutz with my hands," "It's boring repetition of over-paid procedures." Pediatrics is not considered to be intellectual enough; neurology, psychiatry, and pediatrics are all characterized as "too narrow"; family medicine as "too broad."

What Do You Like Most About General Internal Medicine?

Intellectual stimulation and grateful patients are the two aspects that are most enjoyable. Respondents particularly like "interesting cases" and "the problem solving and data interpretation required to make a diagnosis and to treat patients properly."

What Do You Like Least About General Internal Medicine?

Physicians in general internal medicine report low satisfaction rates (36.5 percent say "very satisfied" and 20.3 percent say "dissatisfied").[6] Ten percent of internists originally certified between 1990 and 1995 are no longer working in general internal medicine or one of its subspecialties. A significantly lower proportion of general internists (70 percent) than internal medicine subspecialists (77 percent) were satisfied with their career.[7]

The long and uncertain hours ". . . making it difficult to organize an outside life" is the one frustration cited by almost all respondents. One says, "In a small town the demands placed on your time are substantial; people call frequently at my home." Another respondent believes that "working in an HMO limits my independence."

What Is Your Typical Daily Schedule?

General internal medicine today is, either primarily an office-based practice or a hospitalist practice. There is information on hospitalist medicine in Part 4 of the book. Office based respondents report working from 10 to 12 hours per day with an on-call schedule that varies with the type of practice, that is, if part of a four-person group, you may be on call every fourth night and weekend. A few general internists also spend time making house calls and nursing home visits.

The patients are usually all adults, although one respondent reports caring for teenagers. Many of the internists' patients are elderly and have multiple chronic illnesses. Much of the practice is primary care—only 10 to 15 percent of the daily patient visits are in response to requests for consultations from other physicians. In contrast, subspecialty internists' daily referral visits range from 20 to 45 percent of their total patient visits.[8]

What Abilities and Talents Are Important in General Internal Medicine?

The general internist needs to have "good scientific ability" and "interpersonal skills." Specifically, the ability to be patient is very important: "You need to be persistent in following a case and able to work long hours—you won't make many dumb mistakes nor lose a family's confidence if you are diligent."

What Personality Traits Characterize General Internists?

The traits of thoroughness, constancy, and deliberateness allow the general internist "to persevere through long illnesses." More thoughtful and cautious than active and aggressive, the general internist is characterized as a problem solver and a good listener. A contrast is drawn with surgeons: "Internists sit around and theorize but surgeons like to hurry and get at it."[9]

The Myers-Briggs Type Indicator data predict that those who enjoy direct patient care will choose general internal medicine. Those who prefer the more complex and difficult cases will gravitate to the subspecialties in internal medicine. The general internists' personality traits are similar to those of family physicians whereas the subspecialists' traits are more science-oriented and academic.

What Advice Would You Give a Medical Student Interested in General Internal Medicine?

While in medical school "care for as many patients as you can under skilled supervision. Take extra training in cardiac, pulmonary, and critical care." It is also important to "find out if you like older people since they will be a large part of your practice."

Duffy[10] advocates student interaction "with internists who are seeing healthy adults with preventable problems or adults with serious illness in the rehabilitation and recovery stages."

What Are the Future Challenges to General Internal Medicine?

More than half of the general internists spend most of their practice time in the office setting, especially in urban settings[11-12] with the rise of the hospitalists who are engaged in full-time hospital practice. Those who choose office-based practice will be expected to provide a wider range of services than traditional training programs teach, such as procedural skills, gynecology, psychosocial training, and adolescent health care. Other challenges include governmental regulations—"telling us how to practice"—and the need to keep up with new knowledge that relates to this broad-based specialty.

REFERENCES

1. Vyskocil JJ, Whitney-Merritt K, Milliken JP, McIlroy MA. Medical students' perceptions of the practice of internal medicine. *Acad Med* 1991;66(12):747–748.

2. Coombs RH. *Mastering medicine.* New York: The Free Press, 1978, pp. 188–189.

3. Goodman L. Editorial: Adult (not internal) medicine. *Ann Int Med* 1997;127(9):835–836.

4. Park J, Liner RS. To What Extent is there a Hidden System of Primary Care Provided by Subspecialists? Presentation at the Academy Health Annual Research Meeting, June 2010, information accessed at www.abim.org/research/abstracts/system -of-primary-care.aspx?print December 26, 2010.

5. Anwar RAH. Trends in training: Focus on emergency medicine. *Ann Emer Med* 1980;9:60–71.

6. Leigh JP, Kravitz RL, Schembri M, Samuels SJ,, Mobley S. Physician career satisfaction across specialties. *Arch Intern Med* 2002; 162:1577-1584.

7. Blysma WH, Arnold GK, Fortna GS, Lipner RS. Where have all the general internists gone? *Jour Gen Int Med* 2009; 25(10):1020-1023.

8. *The internist.* Brochure prepared by the Federated Council for Internal Medicine.

9. Wahls TL, Stene RA, Olson KA. General internal medicine practice trends in large multispecialty clinics. *J Gen Int Med* 1991;6(2):103–107.

10. Duffy T. In Wogensen EO. Internal angst. *The New Physician* 1992;41(2):18–23.

11. Saint S, Konrad TR, Golin CE, Welsh DE, Linzer M for the SGIM Career Satisfaction Study Group. Characteristics of general internists who practice only outpatient medicine: Results from the Physician Worklife Study. *Seminars in Medical Practice* 2002;5(1):5-12.

12. Grosso L, Iobst W, Lipner RS, Jacobs C. American Board of Internal Medicine's Workforce Data: Residents, Fellows, and Practicing Physicians. Presented at the AAMC Physician Workforce Research Meeting, May 2010.

Job Values Selections of General Internists

You can complete the questionnaires and obtain your scores for all specialties online at http://www.sdn.net, or compare your job values (as recorded in the Appendix) with the job values of general internists:

General Internists' Choices:	My Choices:
1. Working with my mind	1. _____
2. Independence	2. _____
3. Working with people	3. _____
4. Taking care of people	4. _____

No one chose: Working with my hands

Summary Profile of General Internists   **My Personal Profile**
(derived from questionnaire answers)   **as a General Internist**

They tend to: I tend to: (circle one number)

	Never	Rarely	Sometimes	Frequently	Always
Become bored with repetitive activity	1	2	3	4	5
Like complex problem solving	1	2	3	4	5
Value independence highly	1	2	3	4	5
Be interested in people	1	2	3	4	5
Have good listening skills/interested in listening	1	2	3	4	5
Accept long-term outcomes	1	2	3	4	5
Be thinkers rather than "doers"	1	2	3	4	5
Be thorough and deliberate	1	2	3	4	5
Enjoy long-term relationships with people	1	2	3	4	5
Be good coordinators	1	2	3	4	5

Add total of numbers circled to get your TOTAL SCORE: _____

Transfer score to the Appendix.

General internal medicine

> sounds like me_____

> could be a possibility _____

> doesn't sound like me at all _____

SUBSPECIALTIES IN INTERNAL MEDICINE

There are fellowship programs leading to subspecialty certification in internal medicine: adolescent medicine; advanced heart failure and transplant cardiology; cardiovascular disease; clinical cardiac electrophysiology; critical care medicine; endocrinology, diabetes, and metabolism; gastroenterology; geriatric medicine; hematology; hospice and palliative medicine; infectious disease; medical oncology; nephrology; pulmonary disease; rheumatology; sleep medicine; and sports medicine. Board certification in allergy and immunology can also be achieved through an internal medicine or pediatrics pathway, and information on this specialty is covered separately.

Board certification in internal medicine and successful completion of at two to four years, depending on the specialty, of full-time subspecialty training are prerequisites for application to the written certification examinations for all subspecialties of internal medicine. Certification in more than one subspecialty is not encouraged. However, requirements for dual certification in hematology and in medical oncology have been published and three years of training in these fields is required.

Nearly 60 percent of the physicians who complete three years of internal medicine residency training eventually subspecialize.[1] Even those who don't aim for subspecialty board certification may take an additional year of training in a subspecialty. What factors cause this to happen? One study [2] attributes this to the influence of mentors, lifestyle issues, prestige and financial rewards. Another study [3] showed that residents training in high managed care locations (greater than 30 percent penetration) were more likely not to subspecialize than those from communities with lower managed care penetration.

Internal medicine subspecialists usually have a higher income than general internists. Those subspecialties that offer technological services, such as cardiology and gastroenterology, have been reimbursed by third-party payers to a greater extent than those that offer cognitive services.

Internal medicine subspecialists have a variety of practice options, such as private practice, research, or academics. If you choose private practice, you'll need to be located in a large, highly populated area in order to have the necessary hospital facilities and numbers of people who need your services. If you practice in a less populated setting, it will be necessary to keep current in general medical care in addition to the more specialized areas of your training since there will not be enough patients who need your subspecialty care to do this full time.

REFERENCES

1. Grosso L, Iobst W, Lipner RS, Jacobs C. American Board of Internal Medicine's Workforce Data: Residents, Fellows, and Practicing Physicians. Presented at the AAMC Physician Workforce Research Meeting, May 2010.
2. DeWitt DE, Curtis JR, Burke W. What influences career choices among graduates of a primary care training program? *J Gen Intern Med* 1998;13:257-261.
3. Nelson HD, Matthews AM, Patrizio GR, Cooney TG. Managed care, attitudes and career choices of internal medicine residents. *J Gen Intern Med* 1998;13(1):39-42.

Cardiology

█████ ▌FAST FACTS: ▌█████

Number of fellowship positions matched in 2010 to start in 2011: 475
Competitiveness: Very high
Length of training: 6 years (3 years plus 3 years of an internal medicine residency)
Number of residency programs: 180
Number of residents/fellows in training: 2,429
Number in US Board Certified in Cardiology: 23,760
Number in US Board Certified in Interventional Cardiology; 5,108
Starting median compensation: $267,000
Median compensation for all general cardiologists: $300,000
Median compensation for all invasive cardiologists: $310,500
Average work hours per week: 65

CARDIOLOGY IS CONCERNED WITH DEFECTS AND DISEASES of the cardiovascular system, including the heart, blood vessels, and the circulation of blood through the body.

Those cardiologists who become interested in full-time subspecialization in cardiology—in areas such as pediatric cardiology, nuclear cardiology, or catheterization—usually practice in university hospitals or large medical centers. Cardiologists may seek a certificate of added qualification in clinical cardiac electrophysiology and post-fellowship training in nuclear cardiology and cardiac catheterization.

Invasive cardiologists, who run cardiac-catheterization labs, are among the highest paid physicians and are said to make up three-quarters of all cardiologists. Cardiology is currently a specialty in high demand, especially for those working in the fields of electro-physiology, interventional cardiology and nuclear medicine. [1]

Further Information. The American College of Cardiology, 2400 N Street NW, Washington, DC 20037. Telephone: (800) 253-4636. Internet address: www.acc.org.

A COMPOSITE PICTURE OF THE CARDIOLOGIST
Why Choose Cardiology?
Faculty role models and intellectual challenges attracted the re-spondents to cardiology. One respondent "prefers dealing with life-threatening disease on a day-to-day basis" and performing pro-cedures and, therefore, would not want to practice pediatrics, general medicine, or psychiatry. Hematology is described as "too laboratory oriented and, in practice, too slanted to oncology"; cardiology has "better results of treatment." Respondents prefer patient-oriented spe-cialties with some diversity.

What Do You Like Most About Cardiology?
Satisfaction comes from seeing patients improve, not just in caring for them. Cardiologists report that they like to have a definite diagnosis and be able to "do" something to cure the patient. Also enjoyable are "the technical procedures in the cath lab which involve some manual dexterity." Slightly more than all physicians (42.3 percent), cardiol-ogists report that they are "very satisfied" (43.8 percent); 16.5 percent are "dissatisfied." [2]

What Do You Like Least About Cardiology?
Long hours with "constant pressure with regard to time and small details" are a stressful factor. Respondents all report that they dislike "paperwork."

What Is Your Typical Daily Schedule?

Cardiology respondents work as long as or, in some cases, longer hours than most surgeon respondents. They have a particularly heavy responsibility caring for seriously ill hospitalized patients and report frequent nighttime calls requiring visits to the hospital. In addition, they have office-based practices and evaluate new patients or follow up on known individuals. Even though this is a referral specialty, many patients consider their cardiologist to be their primary care provider since heart disease involves continuing care.

What Abilities and Talents Are Important in Cardiology?

Manual dexterity is important to be able to put in a pacemaker or do cardiac catheterizations. Also you need to be able to "visualize in three dimensions" and "think through the physiology of the heart." It is also necessary to develop "rigorous scientific knowledge, combined with skepticism, clinical intuition, tact and sensitivity, and physical vigor."

What Personality Traits Characterize Cardiologists?

"Most of us are high pressure, Type A prima donnas." One respondent says that ". . . many cardiologists like gadgets."

The Myers-Briggs Type Indicator data indicate that cardiologists enjoy complex problems and are scientifically oriented.

What Advice Would You Give a Medical Student Interested in Cardiology?

Students are advised that the nature of the work is physically exhausting: "Problems can rarely be put off for a long period and often require immediate attention." Also, "Be aware that at this time the specialty is highly procedure-oriented."

On the other hand, "Cardiology has the advantage of offering the mental challenge of physical diagnosis and providing opportunities to perform minor surgical procedures." If you decide to choose cardiology, "be an internist first and a cardiologist second—learn to see the problems of cardiology in their proper perspective."

What Are the Future Challenges to Cardiology?

Almost all respondents saw the challenges in terms of technological and diagnostic advances. A word of warning is sounded, however: "We can do so much but the increasing numbers of older people means that the opportunities to intervene are expanding in an era of limited funds."

Using a rough estimate of workforce needs, a doubling of the number of cardiologists is "necessary" between 2000 and 2050. [3]

REFERENCES

1. Greene J. Surging demand for specialists spur salary hikes. *AMNews* October 22/29, 2001.

2. Leigh JP, Kravitz RL, Schembri M, Samuels SJ,, Mobley S. Physician career satisfaction across specialties. *Arch Intern Med* 2002; 162:1577-1584.

3. ACC 2009 Survey Results and recommendations: Addressing the Cardiology Workforce Crisis. A Report of the ACC Board of Trustees Workforce Task Force. J Am Coll Cardio 2009; 54:1195-1208.

Job Values Selection of Cardiologists

You can complete the questionnaires and obtain your scores for all specialties online at http://www.sdn.net, or compare your job values (as recorded in the Appendix) with the job values of cardiologist respondents below:

Cardiologists' Choices:	My Choices:
1. Working with my mind	1. _____
1. Working with my hands	2. _____
2. Decision making	3. _____
3. Independence	4. _____
3. Working with people	
(there is a tie for first and third place)	

No one chose: Security, sufficient time off, feedback from others

Summary Profile of Cardiologists (derived from questionnaire answers)	My Personal Profile as a Cardiologist				
They tend to:	I tend to: (circle one number)				
	Never	Rarely	Sometimes	Frequently	Always
Become bored with repetitive activity	1	2	3	4	5
Like complex problem solving	1	2	3	4	5
Value independence highly	1	2	3	4	5
Have manual dexterity	1	2	3	4	5
Be interested in people	1	2	3	4	5
Be energetic/have a high energy level	1	2	3	4	5
Be willing to work long hours	1	2	3	4	5
Be uncomfortable with poorly defined problems	1	2	3	4	5
Like gadgets and enjoy technology	1	2	3	4	5
Be serious and determined rather than easy going	1	2	3	4	5

Add total of numbers circled to get your TOTAL SCORE:_____

Transfer score to the Appendix.

Cardiology

sounds like me _____

could be a possibility _____

doesn't sound like me at all _____

Endocrinology and Metabolism

PHYSICIANS WHO SPECIALIZE IN ENDOCRINOLOGY AND ME-
tabolism deal with the diagnosis and treatment of the hormone-pro-
ducing glandular and metabolic systems. There are three categories:
clinical endocrinology, pediatric endocrinology, and reproductive
physiology. Fellowship graduates are in moderate oversupply.

Endocrinologists often earn less than consultants in other areas of
internal medicine, such as in cardiology or gastroenterology, both of
which are more procedure oriented. Many endocrinologists practice in
academic settings in departments of internal medicine, pediatrics, or

obstetrics and gynecology. The majority of endocrinologists practice in large cities (one million or more people).

Further Information. The Endocrine Society, 8401 Connecticut Avenue,, Suite 900, Chevy Chase, MD 20815 . Telephone: (301) 941-0200. Internet address: www.endo-society.org.

A COMPOSITE PICTURE
OF THE ENDOCRINOLOGIST

Why Choose Endocrinology?

Research projects and ward rotations in medical school left a positive impression on the respondents, but most did not make their final choice until residency years. Role models are cited as influential in the decision to be an endocrinologist.

Specialties such as neurology and oncology that deal with incurable patients are not appealing. Neither are specialties that have little patient contact, such as radiology, pathology, and anesthesiology. There is little interest in technical skills, with one respondent who prefers "understanding the basic processes and solving problems."

What Do You Like Most About Endocrinology?

All respondents like the fact that patients have treatable and even curable disorders, and gain a great deal of gratification from positive outcomes. Diagnoses are often precise and management can be readily accomplished. They also enjoy the wide variety of patient problems, the ability to work with and enhance the quality of life in others with chronic illnesses and get to know the patient and family over a long-term relationship, and the experience of "making a correct diagnosis where others have failed." Satisfaction level in this specialty is higher than a national physician sample with 44.9 percent reporting that they are "very satisfied" and only 10.2 percent, "dissatisfied."[1]

What Do You Like Least About Endocrinology?

When patients do not follow recommendations for diet or exercise, the endocrinologist may experience frustration at not being able to influence the course of the disease. Other aspects of endocrinology that are disliked are the amount of nonreimbursed time spent talking to patients, night telephone calls, treatment of advanced complications of diabetes mellitus, the monotony of seeing several patients with the same problem, and those obese patients who ". . . are under the impression their obesity is glandular in nature while the only abnormal glands they actually have are the salivary glands."

What Is Your Typical Daily Schedule?

Endocrinology is primarily an office-based referral practice, but there are hospitalized patients too. The patient population is of all ages and both sexes with the most common problems being diabetes mellitus and thyroid disease. There is long-term continuing care for diabetic patients and telephone calls after hours related to their problems. Those who work in an academic setting report that clinical research activities are pursued on evenings or weekends. Continuing medical education is a necessity because the field is changing rapidly, and respondents spend much time attending conferences and reading journals.

What Abilities and Talents Are Important in Endocrinology?

An endocrinologist should have an interest in basic disease processes and be a good general internist. It is important to have the patience and skill to perform a careful history and physical examination and adopt an organized approach to diagnostic studies.

Because patients "frequently have vague complaints, as many endocrine diagnoses present as vague, nonspecific, generalized complaints and do not categorize very easily," the endocrinologist needs to develop an understanding and supportive attitude toward patients.

What Personality Traits Best Characterize Endocrinologists?

A sympathetic and intellectually curious personality is described by respondents: "Being interested in patients and willing to listen to their complaints along with being willing to sort out large numbers of symptoms and laboratory data to achieve a diagnosis" is characteristic of the endocrinologist. The goal and resulting satisfaction involves being able to get answers and positive results.

What Advice Would You Give a Medical Student Interested in Endocrinology?

"The student should be well grounded in endocrine metabolism and chemistry of the body, knowledgeable about cellular function of the body, and competent in all laboratory procedures to be able to appropriately identify which tests are to be done and when finished, if they have been correctly performed."

It is important to decide if your area of interest in endocrinology is clinical or investigative in order to choose the best training program for your interests.

What Are the Future Challenges to Endocrinology?

The rapid expansion of knowledge in the field of endocrinology in the past 10 to 15 years offers the challenge to bring the advances to the public as quickly as possible. Endocrinology is seen as "an extremely exciting area at present" with improvements in diabetic care, the discovery of new hormones, and a great deal of clinically pertinent research that is intellectually stimulating.

REFERENCE

1. Leigh JP, Kravitz RL, Schembri M, Samuels SJ,, Mobley S. Physician career satisfaction across specialties. *Arch Intern Med* 2002; 162:1577-1584

Job Values Selection of Endocrinologists

You can complete the questionnaires and obtain your scores for all specialties online at http://www.sdn.net, or compare your job values (as recorded in the Appendix) with the job values of endocrinologist respondents below:

Endocrinologists' Choices:	My Choices:
1. Working with my mind	1. _____
2. Taking care of people	2. _____
3. Variety	3. _____
3. Independence	4. _____
(there is a tie for third place)	

No one chose: Good income, prestige, working with my hands, sufficient time off, feedback from others

Summary Profile of Endocrinologists   My Personal Profile as a Endocrinologist (derived from questionnaire answers)

They tend to:	I tend to: (circle one number)				
	Never	Rarely	Sometimes	Frequently	Always
Ask why	1	2	3	4	5
Enjoy taking care of people	1	2	3	4	5
Become bored with repetitive activity	1	2	3	4	5
Like complex problem solving	1	2	3	4	5
Need control over a situation	1	2	3	4	5
Value independence highly	1	2	3	4	5
Enjoy being an "expert"	1	2	3	4	5
Have good listening skills/ interested in listening	1	2	3	4	5
Be uncomfortable with poorly defined problems	1	2	3	4	5
Value organization highly	1	2	3	4	5

Add total of numbers circled to get your TOTAL SCORE: _____

Transfer score to the Appendix.

Endocrinology

   sounds like me _____

   could be a possibility _____

   doesn't sound like me at all _____

Gastroenterology

GASTROENTEROLOGY IS A SUBSPECIALTY OF INTERNAL MEDICINE dealing with the diagnosis and treatment of diseases and disorders related to the digestive system—the esophagus, stomach, gall bladder and biliary tract, liver, pancreas, and small and large intestines. Traditionally, a significant part of gastroenterology has involved the evaluation of psychosomatic complaints as they affect the gastrointestinal tract, but the introduction of fiberoptic peroral endoscopy and colonoscopy has changed the orientation of this specialty making it second only to interventional cardiology of the internal medicine sub-specialties in procedural activities.

The number of self-designated gastroenterologists tripled from 4046 in 1980 to 12,722 in 2008.[1] A mid-1990s workforce study[2] predicted a large oversupply and recommended a 25 to 50 percent decrease in fellowship positions over a five-year period. However, factors such as media publicity about the need for early detection of colon cancer has increased the number of patient visits and consultations requested by other physicians and this specialty now is considered to be undersupplied.

Further Information. The American College of Gastroenterology, P.O. Box 342260, Bethesda MD 20827. Telephone: (301)263-9000. Internet address: www.acg.gi.org.

A COMPOSITE PICTURE OF THE GASTROENTEROLOGIST

Why Choose Gastroenterology?

More than any other internal medicine subspecialists, gastroenterologists begin by trying to be nonspecialists. In 2000 10.9% of their patient care time was spent in primary care activities, more than any of the other internal medicine subspecialists [3]. All the respondents chose this field during their residencies and were positively influenced by gastroenterologists under whom they trained.

Cardiology was a strong second choice for a career, but respondents indicate that there were "too many already in that field." Hospital-based specialties, such as radiology and pathology, have little attraction because they restrict independence and have little patient contact. Surgery and obstetrics are described as "too mechanical and not intellectually challenging enough." One respondent would not want to practice intensive care medicine because "I don't want to be married to a building or practice. I have a hard time refusing care or leaving patients if there is any question of their medical stability."

What Do You Like Most About Gastroenterology?

Procedures, especially endoscopy, are the most enjoyable aspect of gastroenterology because they allow the physician to ". . . markedly alter a patient's evaluation and/or treatment." There is a sense of accomplishment in technical skill in addition to the intellectual challenges of diagnosis. More gastroenterologists are "dissatisfied" (19.5 percent) and less are "very satisfied" (38.5 percent) than all physicians. [4]

What Do You Like Least About Gastroenterology?

"Emotional disorders are hard to manage." Gastroenterologists are frustrated by the "necessity at times to deal with psychophysiological problems without a clear-cut endpoint of success or failure."

What Is Your Typical Daily Schedule?

Half of each 10 to 12 hour day is spent in the hospital, consulting on patients and performing procedures. Most patients are middle aged or older and are referred by primary care physicians. The most common problem is irritable bowel syndrome.

Those gastroenterologists who restrict their practice to their subspecialty (and don't provide primary care for general medical problems) report infrequent after-hours calls: "I take my own call during the week and rarely have a call. I may have one emergency requiring evening or weekend patient care. This is the benefit of doing 100 percent gastroenterology and no primary patient care."

Respondents report attending courses to learn new techniques and continuing medical education meetings to keep abreast of new knowledge in the field more so than many other physicians.

What Abilities and Talents Are Important in Gastroenterology?

Unlike most other areas of internal medicine, it is important to have the technical ability to do procedures, especially endoscopy. Coupled with this is the ability to analyze problems and data.

What Personality Traits Characterize Gastroenterologists?

Gastroenterologists describe themselves as "generally less intense than surgeons, but more intense than internists." In addition, they have a supportive attitude toward patients, and are willing to listen to and tolerate patients with "functional" complaints.

What Advice Would You Give a Medical Student Interested in Gastroenterology?

"There is the danger of thinking about gastroenterology in terms of procedures. It is important to be a good general internist first since 70 percent of the diagnosis is made through the history with the additional 30 percent supplied by the physical examination and testing procedures."

"I suggest that anyone considering gastroenterology as a specialty should also be aware of the need to be a 'total' physician. The gastroenterologist may see patients with symptoms related to cardiology, pulmonary medicine, or infectious disease and must be able to recognize these when caring for the patient."

What Are the Future Challenges to Gastroenterology?

Government intervention in medicine, cost factors, and technological advances are all described as challenges. "Decisions must be made on the appropriate use of new techniques and procedures in diagnosis and therapy, particularly considering cost factors."

REFERENCES

1. Physician Characteristics and Distribution in the United States, 2010, Chicago, American Medical Association, Table 6.2, p. 439.
2. Meyer GS, Jacoby I, Krakauer H, Powell DW, Aurand J, McCardle P. Gastroenterology workforce modeling. *JAMA* 1996;276(9):689–694.
3. Physician Socioeconomic Statistics 2000-2002 edition. American Medical Association, Figure 26, p. 102.
4. Leigh JP, Kravitz RL, Schembri M, Samuels SJ,, Mobley S. Physician career satisfaction across specialties. *Arch Intern Med* 2002; 162:1577-1584.

Job Values Selection of Gastroenterologists

You can complete the questionnaires and obtain your scores for all specialties online at http://www.sdn.net, or compare your job values (as recorded in the Appendix) with the job values of gastroenterologist respondents below:

Gastroenterologists' Choices:	My Choices:
1. Good income	1. _____
1. Working with people	2. _____
2. Independence	3. _____
3. Working with my hands	4. _____
3. Achievement	
(there are ties for first and third place)	

No one chose: Variety, prestige.

Summary Profile of Gastroenterologists (derived from questionnaire answers)	My Personal Profile as a Gastroenterologist				
They tend to:	I tend to: (circle one number)				
	Never	Rarely	Sometimes	Frequently	Always
Value time off	1	2	3	4	5
Like complex problem solving	1	2	3	4	5
Value independence highly	1	2	3	4	5
Have manual dexterity	1	2	3	4	5
Need to see tangible results of their efforts quickly	1	2	3	4	5
Have good listening skills/ interested in listening	1	2	3	4	5
Want a good income	1	2	3	4	5
Be achievers	1	2	3	4	5
Have trouble refusing requests	1	2	3	4	5
Prefer treatable illnesses	1	2	3	4	5

Add total of numbers circled to get your TOTAL SCORE: _____

Transfer score to the Appendix.

Gastroenterology

    sounds like me _____

    could be a possibility _____

    doesn't sound like me at all _____

Hematology

HEMATOLOGY DEALS WITH THE DIAGNOSIS AND TREATMENT of blood disorders. Historically, hematology and oncology were one specialty; they are still combined in most programs. There are only 5 programs training physicians solely in hematology. There is a "critical need for and concern about a pipeline of scientific and clinical investigators." [1] To practice only hematology you may choose an academic setting where you will be involved in clinical work and research. Often in the larger cities, there are hematologists in private practice who specialize in treating blood diseases, such as leukemia. The specialty requires critical thinking and problem-solving skills in caring for patients with certain cancers, genetic diseases and illnesses caused by hospitalization for other conditions. The hematologist is often involved in caring for the critically ill person as well as more common diseases, such as anemia.

Further Information. The American Society of Hematology, 2021 L Street NW, Suite 900, Washington DC 20036. Telephone: (202) 776-0544. Internet address: www.hematology.org.

A COMPOSITE PICTURE OF THE HEMATOLOGIST

Why Choose Hematology?

All the respondents had mentors who figured prominently in their decision to specialize in hematology. One respondent says that he was interested in rheumatology, but didn't have a mentor in the field. The internal medicine subspecialties of infectious disease, nephrology, and endocrinology are described as "too narrow" and cardiology is considered to be "too electronic."

What Do You Like Most About Hematology?

Respondents enjoy this specialty because "It has a wide variety of disorders in a limited field"; "It is a discipline that combines clinical and laboratory diagnosis"; and "There is the opportunity to help people in real need."

What Do You Like Least About Hematology?

Having to deal with terminal illness is the answer given by all the respondents.

What Is Your Typical Daily Schedule?

Hematologists in clinical practice have a similar schedule to other internal medicine subspecialists with patient care in both hospital and office settings. One respondent reports that 75 percent of his patients have malignant disease; the other 25 percent have benign hematology conditions.

What Abilities and Talents Are Important in Hematology?

Knowledge of the broad areas of cell biology, biochemistry, and laboratory technology is important. In addition, you need to have the "clinical acumen at the bedside for diagnosis and management of the patient, including psychosocial aspects of hematologic-oncologic disease." You must learn to be skillful in talking one-to-one with patients about their terminal illnesses. It is particularly important that the hematologist not be "hung up about his or her own mortality."

What Personality Traits Characterize Hematologists?

"Compassionate" is the one word that is cited by all respondents. "Hematologists have the compassion, patience, understanding, and willingness to treat patients and families where terminal illness prevails." They characterize themselves as "relatively nonaggressive" and "meticulous."

What Advice Would You Give a Medical Student Interested in Hematology?

You are advised to "not limit your training to either hematology or oncology if private practice is planned. One must be trained in both and equally so."

Another respondent says, "Pick it if you like the 'hidden wonders' of cell development, cell biology, pathology, genetics, biochemistry, and their relevance to the vast number of problems in patients with primary blood diseases or secondary problems of the blood system."

Above all, you need to have "a genuine desire to help suffering patients, especially those with terminal illnesses."

One word of warning is sounded: Hematology has been squeezed out of clinical practice by oncology. You can still practice hematology if you take two years of training in oncology, but hematology is becoming largely a research field.

What Are the Future Challenges to Hematology?

The challenge expressed by all respondents is to learn more of the causes and treatments of malignant diseases. There are ethical dilemmas emerging in relationship to the roles of the physician, patient, family, and government in terminal care.

REFERENCE

1. Broxmeyer, HE. President's Column: Ensuring a future pipeline of scientific and clinical investigators in hematology. The Hematologist. November/December 2010. Vol 7, No 6, p.

Job Values Selection of Hematologists

You can complete the questionnaires and obtain your scores for all specialties online at http://www.sdn.net, or compare your job values (as recorded in the Appendix) with the job values of hematologist respondents below:

Hematologists' Choices:	My Choices:
1. Taking care of people	1. _____
2. Variety	2. _____
2. Decision making	3. _____
2. Working with people	4. _____
(there is a three-way tie for second place)	

No one chose: Good income, prestige, working with my hands, feedback from others.

Summary Profile of Hematologists (derived from questionnaire answers)	My Personal Profile as a Hematologist				
They tend to:	I tend to: (circle one number)				
	Never	Rarely	Sometimes	Frequently	Always
Pay attention to details	1	2	3	4	5
Enjoy taking care of people	1	2	3	4	5
Want to help people	1	2	3	4	5
Like complex problem solving	1	2	3	4	5
Enjoy being an "expert"	1	2	3	4	5
Act decisively	1	2	3	4	5
Have good listening skills/interested in listening	1	2	3	4	5
Accept long-term outcomes	1	2	3	4	5
Identify with role models	1	2	3	4	5
Be comfortable with their own mortality	1	2	3	4	5

Add total of numbers circled to get your TOTAL SCORE: _____

Transfer score to the Appendix.

Hematology

    sounds like me _____

    could be a possibility _____

    doesn't sound like me at all _____

Infectious Diseases

SUBSPECIALISTS IN INFECTIOUS DISEASES DEAL WITH THE diagnosis and treatment of communicable and contagious diseases. Traditionally, this specialty has been hospital- or university-based and it is only recently that specialists in infectious disease have engaged in private practice. Approximately 43 percent enter academic medicine and 40 percent enter clinical practice in the U.S. [1] The remuneration is less than in more procedure-oriented specialties and it may be necessary to do some general medicine in addition to caring for those with infectious diseases.

This is a rapidly changing field with new medications and new diseases emerging.

Further Information. Infectious Diseases Society of America, 1300 Wilson Boulevard, Suite 300, Arlington, VA 22209. Telephone: (703) 299-0200. Internet address: www.idsociety.org.

A COMPOSITE PICTURE OF THE INFECTIOUS DISEASE PHYSICIAN

Why Choose Infectious Diseases?

A strong influence by role models and the "broad base of internal medicine knowledge required" led respondents to choose infectious diseases as their specialty during residency years.

Such specialties as cardiology and ophthalmology are not appealing because they are "limited to one organ system." Cardiology is seen as "too invasive" and both cardiology and pulmonary medicine have "long hours at night and very sick patients." One specialty that many respondents would not want to practice is pediatrics: "It's too difficult to cope with terminally ill kids and many parents," and "kids can't tell you what's wrong." About psychiatry, one respondent says, "I would be frustrated by the chronicity of the problems and the lack of ability to cure patients permanently."

What Do You Like Most About Infectious Diseases?

The intellectual challenges and the rewards of "curing" people are most enjoyable. It is particularly rewarding to "be able to make the diagnosis" of interesting diseases, affording "lots of respect" from colleagues. Respondents also like dealing with diseases that "may affect any part of the body, are in general treatable, and which may be preventable." The majority of physicians in this specialty are "very satisfied" (50 percent) with only 6.3 percent "dissatisfied." [2]

What Do You Like Least About Infectious Diseases?

All the respondents cite time factors. To be a consultant in an "on demand" specialty makes it hard to control hours. Those in both academic and private practice settings feel that they do not have enough time for all their work—"a great deal of time is required to fully evaluate many cases."

What Is Your Typical Daily Schedule?

The hospital is the primary practice site for infectious disease physicians and the majority of time is spent seeing hospitalized patients. One physician in a private solo practice reports: "I start about 7:30 to 8:00 AM and work in the hospital until 12:30 or 1:00 PM. I see new consults and make follow-up rounds on old consults and hospitalized patients. This involves surgery patients, looking at x-rays, checking on culture results, lab results, etc. I am in the office four afternoons a week, seeing both hospitalized follow-ups and general medicine patients. One afternoon a week I do infection control work at two hospitals. After office hours, I usually eat dinner and then often return to the hospital for several hours to either see more consults or hospitalized patients."

The infectious disease physicians report an erratic "on-call" schedule with the day full of unexpected occurrences. Consultations must be given "on demand" and acute problems develop unexpectedly. They all report serving on hospital infection control committees and being heavily involved with continuing education, to increase their own knowledge base and to teach others.

What Abilities and Talents Are Important in Infectious Diseases?

You need to have "good general medical knowledge" plus a "continual updating of data in the literature, especially antibiotics." The talent to be sensitive to data which are often subtle or missed is important as well as an ability to "note and gather details and approach problems logically."

What Personality Traits Best Characterize Infectious Diseases Physicians?

Respondents describe themselves as "logical thinkers" who are able to integrate complex data. They pay attention to details, often compulsively reviewing records and lab data. Their personality traits make it easy to deal diplomatically with people, including patients, families, and referring physicians. A high energy level allows them to work long hours.

What Advice Would You Give a Medical Student Interested in Infectious Diseases?

All the respondents warn of the long hours and low remuneration, but say that it is potentially "the most rewarding, stimulating, and expanding field in medicine."

Some advise that "infectious diseases is not a wise area to go into for private practice" and that the future of the specialty will be primarily in academic areas.

What Are The Future Challenges to Infectious Diseases?

Three categories are cited: new diseases, which are constantly appearing; new treatments, such as antiviral agents, which are being developed; and new prophylaxis, such as vaccines.

REFERENCES

1.   Subspecialty Careers: Highlights about Careers in Internal Medicine: Infectious Disease. www.acponline.org/medicalstudents/impact/archives/2010/12/subspec/ Accessed January 11, 2011.
2.   Leigh JP, Kravitz RL, Schembri M, Samuels SJ,, Mobley S. Physician career satisfaction across specialties. *Arch Intern Med* 2002; 162:1577-1584.

Job Values Selection of Infectious Diseases Physicians

You can complete the questionnaires and obtain your scores for all specialties online at http://www.sdn.net, or compare your job values (as recorded in the Appendix) with the job values of infectious diseases respondents below:

Infectious Disease Physicians' Choices:	My Choices:
1. Decision making	1. _____
2. Taking care of people	2. _____
3. Variety	3. _____
4. Working with my mind	4. _____

No one chose: Prestige, working with my hands

Summary Profile of Infectious Diseases Physicians (derived from questionnaire answers)	My Personal Profile as an Infectious Diseases Physician				
They tend to:	I tend to: (circle one number)				
	Never	Rarely	Sometimes	Frequently	Always
Ask why	1	2	3	4	5
Pay attention to details	1	2	3	4	5
Enjoy taking care of people	1	2	3	4	5
Like complex problem solving	1	2	3	4	5
Enjoy being an "expert"	1	2	3	4	5
Act decisively	1	2	3	4	5
Accept schedule disruptions	1	2	3	4	5
Be energetic/have a high energy level	1	2	3	4	5
Be uncomfortable with poorly defined problems	1	2	3	4	5
Think logically	1	2	3	4	5

Add total of numbers circled to get your TOTAL SCORE: _____

Transfer score to the Appendix.

Infectious diseases

sounds like me _____

could be a possibility _____

doesn't sound like me at all _____

Medical Oncology

FAST FACTS:

Number of fellowship positions offered in 2011 : 37
Competitiveness: Low , 24.3 % of US grads filled positions
Length of training: 2 years (after completing a 3 year internal medicine residency)
Number of fellowship programs: 12
Number of fellows in training: 116
Number in US Board Certified in Medical Oncology: 11,159
Starting median compensation: $173,000
Median compensation for all physicians in specialty: $210,000
Average work hours per week: 55

MEDICAL ONCOLOGY DEALS WITH THE DIAGNOSIS AND TREATMENT of neoplastic disease. The specialty evolved from hematology and these two fields are combined in nearly all training programs. Cooper's analysis predicts that "between 2005 and 2020, there will be a 14 percent increase in the supply of oncologists and a 55 percent increase in demand, leaving a gap of approximately 4,000 oncologists. It will require a 36 percent increase in the supply of oncologists over that which is projected to meet that demand.[1-2]

Most oncologists enter private practice in a medium- to large-size city. It is not necessary to be affiliated with a cancer center since community hospitals offer support services in oncology.

Further Information. The American Society of Clinical Oncology, 2318 Mill Road, Suite 800, Alexandria, VA 22314. Telephone:(888)282-2552. Internet address: www.asco.org.

A COMPOSITE PICTURE OF THE MEDICAL ONCOLOGIST

Why Choose Medical Oncology?

Although there are no reports of the respondents having family members who were cancer patients, this is often a motivating factor for some oncologists. The respondents found "the challenge of trying to alter the course of patients' illnesses appealing," and all report having been influenced by staff members during residency training in internal medicine. One respondent says, "Oncology is an area many doctors ignore . . . I felt that this was an opportunity for me to do what others thought not worthy of doing and proving that it was worth doing."

Other specialties were unsuitable: Tertiary pediatrics is "too emotionally draining"; family medicine is "too broad for expertise"; and cardiology has "situations that can change dramatically in minutes."

What Do You Like Most About Medical Oncology?

All respondents gave essentially the same answer: "The victories. The times the cancer problem is dealt with successfully—if not curatively, then in providing comfort." When asked "How can you stand doing what you do every day?" one respondent says, "Although most of our patients do not do well, the small percentage of patients who improve and are potentially cured makes it all worth it. The personal comfort that one can give as an oncologist is great and most of our patients appear to genuinely appreciate our efforts regardless of outcome." The majority of physicians in this specialty are "very satisfied" (50.5 percent) with only 11.3 percent "dissatisfied."[3]

What Do You Like Least About Medical Oncology?

Variations on a similar theme are expressed: "The constant exposure to seriously ill patients who expect the impossible from me. Most of our patients invariably die of cancer and a major part of my day is spent dealing with death and dying." "Facing patient care situations where you really can't help—not just death. Death is hard to deal with, but not as bad as unrelievable suffering." "This specialty is one where the physician is constantly reminded of his deficiencies. It is easy to get discouraged after seeing numerous patients fail to respond to treatment in spite of one's best efforts."

What Is Your Typical Daily Schedule?

The average 10- to 12-hour work day is divided between hospital rounds and office visits. One respondent in a four-physician group practice describes his typical day: "I arrive at the hospital at approximately 7:30 AM where I begin to see hospital in-patients. On Monday, Wednesday, and every other Friday I spend approximately two hours in the hospital and the rest of the day is in the office where I continually see patients with a one-hour break for lunch. In-office patients are generally being seen as new consultations or oncology follow-up patients, either for evaluation or to receive in-office chemotherapy. On an average day 20 to 25 patients are seen, 90 percent of whom have cancer. On Tuesday and Thursday I spend the entire day in the hospital where I see all of my hospital patients and also my associates' patients (they see most of my in-hospital patients on Monday, Wednesday, and Friday when I am in the office) and offer consultations on hospitalized patients referred by other specialists."

Oncologists often are called upon to serve on community boards of directors for organizations such as Hospice and the American Cancer Society.

What Abilities and Talents Are Important in Medical Oncology?

You need to develop the ability to deal with your own feelings about death and dying and help people who are in crisis situations. It is important to maintain an optimistic attitude in addition to being honest and empathic. Psychosocial skills need to be attained to deal most effectively with patients and their families. It is particularly important for the physician to have interests and support systems outside of medicine so as to avoid possible burnout.

What Personality Traits Best Characterize Medical Oncologists?

Oncologists have "a willingness to try things with small chances of reward." They described themselves as "optimistic," "able to communicate easily with patients and their families," and "patient in the face of uncertainty about the outcome of treatment."

What Advice Would You Give a Medical Student Interested in Medical Oncology?

"This is a rapidly changing field in which, hopefully, successes will be more frequently encountered." Specifically, "The student interested in this specialty should be one who can handle defeat graciously. He must be willing to 'work on a small margin.' Any student who enjoys close patient contact and making crucial life and death decisions would feel at home in this specialty."

What Are the Future Challenges to Medical Oncology?

Finding cures and better treatments for cancers is the challenge in medical oncology, but all the respondents say that this is a slow process and "probably not a reality in my lifetime."

REFERENCES

1. Hortobagyi GN. A Shortage of Oncologists? The American Society of Clinical Oncology Workforce Study. *Jour of Clin Onc* April 20, 2007;25(12):1468-1469.
2. Erikson C, Salsberg E, Forte G, et al: Future supply and demand for oncologists: Challenges to assuring access to oncology services. *J Onc Pract* November 2008; 4(6): 300.
3. Leigh JP, Kravitz RL, Schembri M, Samuels SJ, Mobley S. Physician career satisfaction across specialties. *Arch Intern Med* 2002; 162:1577-1584.

Job Values Selection of Medical Oncologists

You can complete the questionnaires and obtain your scores for all specialties online at http://www.sdn.net, or compare your job values (as recorded in the Appendix)with the job values of medical oncologist respondents below:

Medical Oncologists' Choices:	My Choices:
1. Taking care of people	1. _____
2. Decision making	2. _____
2. Independence	3. _____
2. Working with people	4. _____
(there is a three-way tie for second place)	

No one chose: Prestige

Summary Profile of Medical Oncologists (derived from questionnaire answers)	My Personal Profile as a Medical Oncologist				
They tend to:	I tend to: (circle one number)				
	Never	Rarely	Sometimes	Frequently	Always
Enjoy taking care of people	1	2	3	4	5
Want to help people	1	2	3	4	5
Value independence highly	1	2	3	4	5
Act decisively	1	2	3	4	5
Have good listening skills/ interested in listening	1	2	3	4	5
Tolerate the unknown	1	2	3	4	5
Accept long-term outcomes	1	2	3	4	5
Be comfortable with their own mortality	1	2	3	4	5
Be optimistic	1	2	3	4	5
Be able to handle defeat graciously	1	2	3	4	5

Add total of numbers circled to get your TOTAL SCORE: _____

Transfer score to the Appendix.

Medical oncology

sounds like me _____

could be a possibility _____

doesn't sound like me at all _____

Nephrology

FAST FACTS:

Number of fellowship positions offered in 2011: 380

Competitiveness: Low, 24.2 % filled by US grads

Length of training: 2 years (after completing a 3 year internal medicine residency)

Number of fellowship programs: 146

Number of fellows in training: 911

Number in US Board Certified in Nephrology: 8,565

Starting median compensation: $200,000

Median compensation of all physicians in specialty: $260,000

Average work hours per week: 51

NEPHROLOGY IS CONCERNED WITH THE DIAGNOSIS AND treatment of renal (kidney) disease and related problems. The demand for nephrologists' services will probably grow with the aging population. Nephrologists usually practice in partnerships or groups with other nephrologists because care of patients with renal disease often involves intensive and "around-the-clock" professional service.

Further Information. The American Society of Nephrology, 1725 I Street, NW, Suite 510, Washington DC 20006. Telephone: (202)659-0599. www.asn-online.org

A COMPOSITE PICTURE OF THE NEPHROLOGIST
Why Choose Nephrology?

Some respondents were attracted to nephrology as a new specialty: "In 1958, nephrology was an unknown specialty and there were many challenges." One respondent became interested in medical school while working on a research project dealing with the kidney. Another found appealing "the challenge of working with very ill patients."

Nephrologist respondents considered choosing the specialties of surgery, pediatrics, general internal medicine, hematology, or infectious diseases but did not find them to be as intellectually challenging as nephrology. Gastroenterology is characterized as "becoming all procedure-oriented" and endocrinology "offered much the same as nephrology." They would not want to practice psychiatry because ". . . I would not want to deal with patients' personal problems exclusively"; nor oncology "due to the constant loss of patients"; nor pathology and radiology because there were "no live patients."

What Do You Like Most About Nephrology?

Two aspects are cited: the dramatic clinical responses possible and the diagnostic and therapeutic problem-solving process. "It is one of the few specialties where application of its treatment principles is absolutely life-saving. Therefore, it offers real gratification to the physician. In addition, I feel that caring for the renal patient and all the complications is most challenging and a dynamic form of medicine." Forty six percent of physicians in this specialty are "very satisfied" with only 9 percent "dissatisfied." [1]

What Do You Like Least About Nephrology?

Responses fall into two areas: the increasing governmental regulations and the strain of caring for very ill patients: "the intrusion of bureaucratic planning, payment, review and federal control organizations" and "the frequent psychological problems and the large number of chronically debilitated patients."

What Is Your Typical Daily Schedule?

Some nephrologists spend most of their time supervising a dialysis unit, either independent or a part of a hospital. Others do not offer dialysis care and divide their time between consultations on hospitalized patients and seeing patients in a private office. Respondents all report a 10- to 12-hour day with an increasing amount of administrative paperwork related to federal and state regulations. On-call schedules vary with the type of practice arrangements and there are numerous hospital meetings, especially in connection with the dialysis unit.

A study[2] reported that 90 percent of respondents provided primary care to their dialysis patients. Older and more experienced physicians were most likely to provide this type of care.

What Abilities and Talents Are Important in Nephrology?

Stamina, both physical and emotional, is important for a nephrologist. It is especially important to develop the ability to "work well with patients and their families and be empathic to their long-standing, chronic illness." Also needed is the perseverance to deal with long-term management and the ability "to not be depressed or unrealistic about frequent failures."

What Personality Traits Best Characterize Nephrologists?

Nephrologists most often describe themselves as "aggressive," "compulsive about every detail," "decisive," "energetic," and "outgoing." They particularly see themselves as "having a positive attitude about the seriously ill patient."

What Advice Would You Give a Medical Student Interested in Nephrology?

Students are advised to have a rotation with a nephrologist away from the medical center because the clinical experience is said to be different from working with hospitalized patients.

Some respondents are discouraged about the future satisfactions in nephrology as a specialty, and warn of the increasingly complex regulations and "constant abuse by the bureaucrats on the pretense that renal physicians are overcompensated."

What Are the Future Challenges to Nephrology?

Cost and ethical considerations figure prominently in nephrology: "We must contain costs and provide excellent care in the light of arbitrary government decisions." In addition to the social challenges, there are medical challenges—"innovations in the treatment of renal failure," "equipment refinement," and "perfecting kidney transplants."

REFERENCES

1. Leigh JP, Kravitz RL, Schembri M, Samuels SJ, Mobley S. Physician career satisfaction across specialties. *Arch Intern Med* 2002; 162:1577-1584.
2. Bender FH, Holley JL. Most nephrologists are primary care providers for chronic dialysis patients: Results of a national survey. *Am J Kidney Dis* 1996;28(1):67–71.

Job Values Selection of Nephrologists

You can complete the questionnaires and obtain your scores for all specialties online at http://www.sdn.net, or compare your job values (as recorded in the Appendix) with the job values of nephrologist respondents below:

Nephrologists' Choices:	My Choices:
1. Variety	1. _____
2. Working with my mind	2. _____
2. Taking care of people	3. _____
2. Independence	4. _____
(there is a three-way tie for second place)	

No one chose: Good income, prestige, feedback from others

Summary Profile of Nephrologists   My Personal Profile as a Nephrologist (derived from questionnaire answers)

They tend to:	I tend to: (circle one number)				
	Never	Rarely	Sometimes	Frequently	Always
Pay attention to details	1	2	3	4	5
Enjoy taking care of people	1	2	3	4	5
Like complex problem solving	1	2	3	4	5
Value independence highly	1	2	3	4	5
Be outgoing	1	2	3	4	5
Act decisively	1	2	3	4	5
Be adventurous/like challenges	1	2	3	4	5
Accept long-term outcomes	1	2	3	4	5
Be energetic/have a high energy level	1	2	3	4	5
Be persevering	1	2	3	4	5

Add total of numbers circled to get your TOTAL SCORE: _____

Transfer score to the Appendix.

Nephrology

    sounds like me _____

    could be a possibility _____

    doesn't sound like me at all _____

Pulmonary Disease

FAST FACTS:

Number of fellowship positions in Pulmonary Disease offered in 2011: 21
Competitiveness: Low (4.8% filled by US grads)
Length of training: 2 years (after completing a 3 year internal medicine residency)
Number of fellowship programs: 21
Number of fellows in training: 76
Number in US Board Certified in Pulmonary Diseases: 11,945
Starting median compensation: $200,000
Median compensation for all physicians in specialty: $ 303,000
Average work hours per week: 55

PULMONOLOGISTS, OR CHEST PHYSICIANS AS THEY ARE SOME-times called, diagnose and treat diseases of the respiratory system. They may engage in private practice or be employed by hospitals to work in a variety of settings including a respiratory therapy department, pulmonary function laboratory, or intensive care unit. There are also opportunities for full-time practice in an occupational medicine setting. Training in critical care is integrated into most pulmonary fellowship programs. There are 122 programs with 417 positions offered in 2011 in a joint pulmonary critical care fellowship. The competitiveness is low with 45.6 percent US grads filling these positions.

The number of self-designated pulmonologists has almost tripled since 1980. With the aging population, there is concern that there will be serious shortage of intensive care physicians and pulmonologists.

Further Information. The American College of Chest Physicians, 3300 Dundee Road, Northbrook, IL 60062. Telephone: (847) 498-1400. Internet address: www.chestnet.org.

The American Thoracic Society, 61 Broadway, New York, NY 10006. Telephone: (212) 315-8600. Internet address: www.thoracic.org.

A COMPOSITE PICTURE OF THE PULMONOLOGIST

Why Choose Pulmonary Disease?

Respondents were attracted to this relatively new specialty during their internal medicine residency years. Some cite the influence of a "dynamic teacher"; others viewed this field as combining "the surgical-type excitement of invasive procedures and critical care with the internal medicine type of intellectual stimulation."

Surgery was not selected as a career because it was seen as lacking cerebral skills: "Pneumonectomy in 1933 and now are identical, largely a technical skill." One respondent felt it was important to have a procedure unique to the specialty he chose and, although he enjoyed infectious diseases, it did not meet this criterion. Respondents would not want to practice psychiatry because it is "too hard to listen and not do" or general medicine which they believed was "impossible to do well."

What Do You Like Most About Pulmonary Disease?

The respondents have a problem-solving orientation and most enjoy "the physiologic-medical correlations." One says, "I like to investigate unknown chest lesions and treat reversible lung disease." Satisfaction is reported to be low with only 33.3 percent of pulmonologists "very satisfied" and 17.9 percent "dissatisfied." [1]

What Do You Like Least About Pulmonary Disease?

For some the pressure of critical care is stressful and all report the high death rate to be one of the unfavorable aspects of the practice.

One respondent finds "office outpatients" the least liked aspect of this specialty.

What Is Your Typical Daily Schedule?

There is a great deal of variation in the respondents' daily schedules. Some spend most of their days in office-based practice; others rarely see patients outside of the hospital. Time in the hospital may be spent making rounds in the intensive care unit; doing procedures, such as bronchoscopies; or supervising the pulmonary function laboratory. Some do full- or part-time critical care. Pulmonologists report that they are involved in in-service training for respiratory therapists and serve on many hospital committees. The most commonly seen clinical problems are asthma, chronic obstructive pulmonary disease, and lung cancer.

What Abilities and Talents Are Important in Pulmonary Disease?

Some manual dexterity to perform procedures, and mechanical aptitude to understand pulmonary function are necessary. As in all referral specialties, it is helpful to develop skills in communicating with other health professionals as well as in dealing with patients and their families.

What Personality Traits Best Characterize Pulmonologists?

Intellectual curiosity and emotional stability are most often cited as personality traits of pulmonologists. The Myers-Briggs Type Indicator data report that this specialty seems to attract physicians who like complex problems and are tough-minded and objective.

What Advice Would You Give a Medical Student Interested in Pulmonary Disease?

While in medical school it is helpful to take a radiology rotation. It is important to have a good background in physiology and infectious disease and "be able to apply them to the science and art of medicine."

What Are the Future Challenges to Pulmonary Disease?

The scientific advances in better treatment of lung disease and asthma as well as "social changes to prevent disease due to cigarette smoking and industry" are future challenges. The recent genetic advances in cystic fibrosis, lung cancer, and asthma are likely to have clinical implications in the near future.

REFERENCE

1. Leigh JP, Kravitz RL, Schembri M, Samuels SJ, Mobley S. Physician career satisfaction across specialties. *Arch Intern Med* 2002; 162:1577-1584.

Job Values Selection of Pulmonologists

You can complete the questionnaires and obtain your scores for all specialties online at http://www.sdn.net, or compare your job values (as recorded in the Appendix) with the job values of pulmonologist respondents below:

Pulmonologists' Choices:	My Choices:
1. Decision making	1. _____
1. Working with my mind	2. _____
1. Taking care of people	3. _____
1. Variety	4. _____
(there is a four-way tie for first place)	

No one chose: Security, independence, prestige, working with my hands, sufficient time off, feedback from others

Summary Profile of Pulmonologists (derived from questionnaire answers)   **My Personal Profile as a Pulmonologist**

They tend to:	I tend to: (circle one number)				
	Never	Rarely	Sometimes	Frequently	Always
Ask why	1	2	3	4	5
Pay attention to details	1	2	3	4	5
Enjoy taking care of people	1	2	3	4	5
Become bored with repetitive activity	1	2	3	4	5
Like complex problem solving	1	2	3	4	5
Have manual dexterity	1	2	3	4	5
Act decisively	1	2	3	4	5
Have mechanical aptitude	1	2	3	4	5
Be objective	1	2	3	4	5
Be "doers" rather than talkers	1	2	3	4	5

Add total of numbers circled to get your TOTAL SCORE:_____

Transfer score to the Appendix.

Pulmonary disease

sounds like me_____

could be a possibility_____

doesn't sound like me at all_____

Rheumatology

FAST FACTS:

Number of fellowship positions offered in 2011: 184

Competitiveness: Low (43.5% US grads matched)

Length of training: 2 years (after completing a 3 year internal medicine residency)

Number of fellowship programs: 108

Number of fellows in training: 288

Number in US Board Certified in Rheumatology: 4,968

Staring median compensation: $195,000

Median compensation for all physicians in specialty: $ 250,000

Average work hours per week: 51

RHEUMATOLOGISTS DIAGNOSE AND TREAT RHEUMATIC DISEASES and musculoskeletal problems. This specialty had four years of explosive growth with the number of American College of Rheumatology members who designated rheumatology as their primary activity doubling from 916 in 1975 to 1884 in 1979.[1] Workforce analysis[2] reports that even with approximately 5,000 physicians in the specialty, demand in 2025 is projected to exceed supply because of the aging population, physician retirements, and flat supply. Most rheumatologists are in private practice in urban areas. About 25 percent are in full-time academic positions.

Further Information. The American College of Rheumatology, 2200 Lake Boulevard NE, Atlanta, GA 30319. Telephone: (404) 633-3777. Internet address: www.rheumatology.org.

A COMPOSITE PICTURE OF THE RHEUMATOLOGIST
Why Choose Rheumatology?

The experience of doing research in this field and the influence of physician advisors led most of the respondents to choose rheumatology as a specialty. Another chose this field because "At the time I was in residency, there were few people who knew much about rheumatology-related disorders, and the situation for the patients seemed so hopeless. In addition, the illnesses on the rheumatology service seemed very complex and challenging to diagnose and treat."

Respondents say they would not want to practice surgery which "lacks intellectual challenge"; obstetrics and gynecology had "erratic hours [and was] surgically oriented, unisex"; or oncology which has a "high mortality" rate. One respondent considered cardiology but "enjoyed the broader scope of rheumatology where diseases tend to be multisystem, demanding more skill and ability to manage." Hematology and neurology are characterized as "too intellectual and esoteric."

What Do You Like Most About Rheumatology?

It is gratifying to see even small gains: "A chronic, debilitating disorder often takes more courage to face than death itself. The smallest bit of improvement is so gratifying to the patient and hence to me. You can almost always do something to improve the situation." Another cites the diagnostic challenges and therapeutic dilemmas as positive factors in this specialty. Rheumatologists report similar numbers as "very satisfied" (42.6 percent) and "dissatisfied"(18 percent) to the national median numbers for all physicians.[3]

What Do You Like Least About Rheumatology?

Rheumatologists have few disatisfactions, citing only administrative tasks and communication problems with patients, stresses that occur in all other specialties.

What Is Your Typical Daily Schedule?

Rheumatology is largely an office-based practice. Some respondents report that they care for, on the average, only one hospitalized patient per day, although they may provide consultations to other specialty physicians. Respondents report working from 9 to 10 hours daily, seeing patients of all ages who have usually been referred by family physicians or general internists. After-hours call is not demanding. A strong commitment to hospital committee work and teaching is reported by all respondents.

What Abilities and Talents Are Important in Rheumatology?

All respondents emphasize the need to develop patience, understanding, compassion, and thoroughness. "You are dealing with people who have chronic diseases which are not curable for the most part. Their diseases cause pain and disability. You can help them, but you have to determine how the disease has affected the patient and how the patient has affected the disease."

What Personality Traits Best Characterize Rheumatologists?

Rheumatologists view themselves as intellectual, compassionate, patient, practical, and compulsive. "It is important to have a personality that can withstand personal frustration and focus attention on the patient's care and comfort."

What Advice Would You Give a Medical Student Interested in Rheumatology?

While in medical school, you are advised to "get a good background in biochemistry, immunology, and radiology." Another respondent says, "Students should obtain training in internal medicine, neurology, orthopedics, psychiatry, orthotics-prosthetics, and rehabilitative medicine."

"If you read, investigate, and are curious and critical, then rheumatology may be for you."

What Are the Future Challenges to Rheumatology?

Rheumatologists see themselves as working in a "crisis-oriented health care system" and say that the challenge is to "educate the public to seek attention early to avoid irreversible joint destruction." Scientific challenges include "determining the causes of virtually all the diseases we deal with in hopes of providing more effective therapy."

REFERENCES

1. Schumacher HR, Lockshin M. Manpower and fellowship education in rheumatology, 1980. *Arthritis Rheum* 1981;24(9):1168–1172.
2. Deal CL, Hooker R, Harrington T, et al. The United States rheumatology workforce: supply and demand, 2005-1025. *Arthritis Rheum* 2007; 56(3):722-729.
3. Leigh JP, Kravitz RL, Schembri M, Samuels SJ, Mobley S. Physician career satisfaction across specialties. *Arch Intern Med* 2002; 162:1577-1584.

Job Values Selection of Rheumatologists

You can complete the questionnaires and obtain your scores for all specialties online at http://www.sdn.net, or compare your job values (as recorded in the Appendix) with the job values of rheumatologist respondents below:

Rheumatologists' Choices:	My Choices:
1. Decision making	1. _____
2. Working with my mind	2. _____
3. Taking care of people	3. _____
4. Variety	4. _____

No one chose: Good income, working with people, working with my hands, feedback from others

Summary Profile of Rheumatologists (derived from questionnaire answers)	My Personal Profile as a Rheumatologist				
They tend to:	I tend to: (circle one number)				
	Never	Rarely	Sometimes	Frequently	Always
Ask why	1	2	3	4	5
Pay attention to details	1	2	3	4	5
Enjoy taking care of people	1	2	3	4	5
Like complex problem solving	1	2	3	4	5
Prefer a planned schedule	1	2	3	4	5
Act decisively	1	2	3	4	5
Have good listening skills/ interested in listening	1	2	3	4	5
Accept long-term outcomes	1	2	3	4	5
Be thinkers rather than "doers"	1	2	3	4	5
Find satisfaction in small gains	1	2	3	4	5

Add total of numbers circled to get your TOTAL SCORE:_____

Transfer score to the Appendix.

Rheumatology

sounds like me_____

could be a possibility_____

doesn't sound like me at all_____

Medical Genetics

FAST FACTS:

Number of fellowship positions offered in 2011: 53

Competitiveness level: Low (15.1% filled by US grads)

Total number of fellowship programs: 36

Total number of residents in training: 84

Number of Combined Internal Medicine/Genetics residency programs in 2011: 7

Number of Combined Pediatrics/Genetics residency programs in 2011: 11

Number of Combined Maternal Fetal Medicine/Genetics residency programs in 2011: 12

Competitiveness: Low

Length of training: 4 years (two year program after two years of a residency in another specialty area)

Number in US Board Certified in Medical Genetics: 108

Median compensation for all physicians in specialty: lower than $194,400 reported for all MDs

Average work hours per week: 49

APPROVED AS A BONA FIDE CLINICAL SPECIALTY AND THE twenty-fourth member of the American Board of Medical Specialties in 1993, medical genetics has evolved over the past 40 years from a basic science to a clinical discipline that many believe will become a factor in most patient encounters. It is predicted that a "revolution in health care delivery" will result in physicians' increasingly using genetic screening and testing to determine a patient's individual susceptibility to diseases.[1] The key to the integration of medical genetics into the medical practice of all physicians is the basic family history. In addition, as family physician A. Patrick Jonas, M.D., says, "Genetics should bring the medical profession together . . . there isn't a geneticist who can come in and deal with my (individual) patients. Just the same, I can't do what the geneticist does."[1]

Residency Information. Two years of residency training in another medical specialty is the norm for acceptance into a two-year medical genetics residency program. Most medical geneticists have initial training in pediatrics, internal medicine, or obstetrics and gynecology. Some programs have fellowships, but the number of trainees in each program is small.

Board Certification. Medical genetics has become increasingly subspecialized. Both M.D. and Ph.D. geneticists are eligible to seek certification from the American Board of Medical Genetics. Certificates are available in clinical biochemical genetics, clinical cytogenetics, clinical genetics (for M.D.'s), clinical molecular genetics, and Ph.D. medical genetics. An additional year of training is required for certification in molecular genetic pathology.

Supply and Projections. The number of physician medical geneticists is small; approximately 800 physicians are members of the American College of Medical Genetics. All indications are that this is a growing specialty, but it is unclear how many medical geneticists are needed.

Economic Status and Types of Practice. Full-time opportunities for physician medical geneticists are primarily in academic and research centers. Salary negotiations usually are based on the qualifications of the individual.

Further Information. American College of Medical Genetics, 7220 Wisconsin Ave., Suite 300, Bethesda, MD 20814. Telephone: (301)718-9603. Internet address: www.acmg.net. At the website www.ashg.org/genetics/ashg/pubs/tpguide/grad_training.shtml there is the

Graduate Training Programs Guide, a reference source for medical students to get information on all residency programs in this specialty.

A COMPOSITE PICTURE OF THE MEDICAL GENETICIST

Why Choose Medical Genetics?

A personal family experience with inherited disease led to a career in medical genetics for one respondent. Another was "drawn to it during medical school because of my interest in the molecular basis of disease." A residency in internal medicine and research at the National Institutes of Health led another to an academic leadership position.

Also considered as career paths were internal medicine, pediatrics, or obstetrics and gynecology, but the focus was "too broad."

What Do You Like Most About Medical Genetics?

The "scientific-basis" and the "long-term relationship with patients" are appealing. In addition, respondents enjoy working with families as a unit. They find it satisfying to educate other physicians, especially those in primary care, to "be suspicious" and "to ask questions about family history."

What Do You Like Least About Medical Genetics?

The greatest frustration is understanding a disease but not being able to treat it. The uncertainty of when a disease will manifest itself in a family member causes personal concern as "high-burden diagnoses" are made.

What Is Your Typical Daily Schedule?

The time spent in clinical care is primarily on an outpatient basis with a patient mix of about 25 percent adults and 75 percent children. For hospitalized patients, medical geneticists fill the role of consultant and do not have their own hospital service. However, they do have "on-call" schedules for hospital responsibility. There is a varying division of time between clinical and research activities, depending on the personal interests of the medical geneticist.

What Abilities and Talents Are Important in Medical Genetics?

The ability to listen to patients and communicate with them and their family members is imperative in medical genetics. "Up to a third of patients I see have been on the Web to access and handle up-to-date information; so our interactions are often a two-way sharing of data, and I need to be open to learning from my patients."

"We do a lot of risk counseling requiring a pattern-recognition skill and visual memory."

What Personality Traits Best Characterize Medical Geneticists?

"Scholarly" and "introverted" are answers given. Depending upon the career path chosen, a medical geneticist can spend more time in clinical care or in research. Personality factors will be involved in making this choice, with those who prefer to work alone and look for possibilities often seeking research settings and those who prefer patient–family–health care team interaction often pursuing a clinical practice.

What Advice Would You Give a Medical Student Interested in Medical Genetics?

"Do a rotation to see the day-to-day life of the medical geneticist." The summer between the first and second year of medical school is suggested as a good time to explore this interest.

What Are the Future Challenges to Medical Genetics?

Ethical challenges are many. The most often cited is confidentiality, with an AMA survey finding that 68 percent of respondents feared use of their genetic test results by employers or insurers against them.[2]

The financing of medical genetics is a challenge. The value of genetics services on preventive initiatives and a subsequent reduction in potential health care costs should be considered in reimbursement decisions. [3] The cost of testing an individual for even one disease, such as breast cancer genes, is in excess of $2000. The question of who pays is unanswered.[2]

On the other hand, Rakatansky[4] warns that "indiscriminate genetic testing may produce information that will provoke inappropriate medical intervention." He also advises that we should "slow down the application of technology until we have the guidance systems to predict the hazards of its use." Physicians are encouraged to lead the effort to analyze and discuss the results of genetic manipulation.

REFERENCES

1. Mitka M. Changing histories. *Amer Med News* 1998;41(19):17–20.
2. Mitka M. Genetics research already touching your practice. *Amer Med News* 1998;41(13):3,58–59.
3. McKusick VA. Genetics moves into the medical mainstream. *JAMA* 2001;286(18):2322–2323.
4. Rakatansky H. Future of genetics: Watch to avoid Titanic mistakes. *Amer Med News* 1998;41(14):28.

Job Values Selection of Medical Geneticists

You can complete the questionnaires and obtain your scores for all specialties online at http://www.sdn.net, or compare your job values (as recorded in the Appendix) with the job values of medical geneticist respondents below:

Medical Geneticists' Choices:	My Choices:
1. Working with my mind	1. _____
2. Taking care of people	2. _____
3. Working with people	3. _____
4. Creativity	4. _____

No one chose: Good income, working with my hands, sufficient time off, feedback from others.

Summary Profile of Medical Geneticists (derived from questionnaire answers)	My Personal Profile as a Medical Geneticist				
They tend to:	I tend to: (circle one number)				
	Never	Rarely	Sometimes	Frequently	Always
Ask why	1	2	3	4	5
Pay attention to details	1	2	3	4	5
Enjoy taking care of people	1	2	3	4	5
Become bored with repetitive activity	1	2	3	4	5
Like complex problem solving	1	2	3	4	5
Enjoy being an "expert"	1	2	3	4	5
Have good listening skills/ interested in listening	1	2	3	4	5
Be uncomfortable with poorly defined problems	1	2	3	4	5
Value organization highly	1	2	3	4	5
Have interest in the basic science of medicine	1	2	3	4	5

Add total of numbers circled to get your TOTAL SCORE:_____

Transfer score to the Appendix.

Medical genetics

sounds like me_____

could be a possibility_____

doesn't sound like me at all_____

Neurological Surgery

NEUROLOGICAL SURGERY IS CONCERNED WITH THE CENTRAL, peripheral, and autonomic nervous systems and involves diagnosis and, frequently, surgical treatment.

Although considered to be a subspecialty of surgery, the traditional base of neurological surgery is in the laboratory. Early practitioners are described as having been not only "technically skillful surgeons," but also, "in many respects, clinical neurophysiologists." They are depicted as: "During their careers they shuttled between their experimental laboratories, clinical wards, and operating theaters seeing problems, asking questions, and designing appropriate investigative techniques for their resolution."[1]

Residency Information. Before entering a neurological surgery training program, you must complete 12 months of general surgery, which is then followed by five years of a neurological surgery residency.

In 2009 neurological surgery switched to the National Residency Matching Program instead of using its own matching program as it had done in the past. One residency director looks for "an interest in neurology, surgery, and research" in residency applicants. He strongly believes that "personal recommendations to individuals known in other departments are *much* more potent than standard letters of recommendation." It should be noted that "most programs have 25 to 30 good applicants for each position."

Board Certification. To be eligible to take the written examination for certification by the American Board of Neurological Surgery you must complete a postgraduate year-one plus five years in an accredited neurosurgery residency program. The oral examination can be taken after two years of practice.

Supply and Projections. As is the case with the other surgical subspecialties, neurological surgery grew in numbers: American Medical Association (AMA) data show an increase of 33 percent from 1980 to 1996, compared with 38 percent for orthopaedic surgeons, and 11 percent for general surgeons. AMA data show that neurosurgery is continuing to grow.[2]

Economic Status and Types of Practice. Neurosurgeons' incomes are in the higher ranges of surgical subspecialists, but their professional liability insurance premiums are more costly than most other physicians. The majority are engaged in private fee-for-service practices in medium- to large-size cities.

Further Information. The American Association of Neurological Surgeons, 5550 Meadowbrook Drive, Rolling Meadows, IL 60008. Telephone: (888) 566-2267. Internet address: www.neurosurgery.org. There is a student section on the website with a link to information on residencies in the specialty.

A COMPOSITE PICTURE OF THE NEUROLOGICAL SURGEON

Why Choose Neurological Surgery?

The majority of respondents made their career choice of neurological surgery while they were in medical school and all note the influence of a strong role model. One respondent was drawn to neurological surgery as a career because of ". . . the highly technical aspects of the surgical procedures, the level of responsibility and weighty decisions that had to be made regarding the patient care, the anatomical basis of the particular discipline, and the lifestyle which was one of intense activity."

Respondents considered other surgical specialties—"I have a surgical personality (a doer)"—but found them deficient for various reasons. Cardiac surgery was "not intellectual enough, too much emphasis on pure technique"; otolaryngology and ophthalmology were "not challenging enough." One respondent who did not want to be a general surgeon believed that the field is "fading out of existence and specialties will become dominant." Neurosurgeon respondents would not want to practice psychiatry which was "too slow, too unscientific, too few people helped." These same respondents believed neurology lacked a "definitive treatment of patients" and a comment for internal medicine was: "I would be quite frustrated having to spend most of my day in an office and not having the ability to utilize my hands in a surgical subspecialty."

What Do You Like Most About Neurological Surgery?

"The technical aspects of surgery and the immediate feedback from a surgical result" were given as favorable aspects—the same factors respondents cite in other surgical specialties. Neurosurgeons seem to enjoy "sorting out difficult problems."

Another respondent says, "Neurological surgery has a relatively high prestige factor and the fact that the discipline is relatively mysterious to most other practitioners of medicine makes it somewhat more enticing." Forty seven percent of neurosurgeons surveyed in a national study [3] reported being "very satisfied" and 15.2% were "dissatisfied."

What Do You Like Least About Neurological Surgery?

Answers can be divided into two categories. A few of the respondents cite the "increasing burden of paperwork" and "socioeconomic considerations"; the rest are summarized by this answer: "The least appealing aspect of the work relates to the complications of neurological illness. The central and peripheral nervous system, of all the organ systems, is the least able to repair itself. Thus, complications of surgical procedures and complications of the illness produce devastating consequences which are slow to resolve and produce extreme dependency on the part of the patient. I would say that this is an extremely important factor to consider before selecting neurological surgery as a career goal."

What Is Your Typical Daily Schedule?

Neurological surgeons work long hours, all reporting 12 to 14 hours daily with an early morning start. In this time, they will make hospital rounds, engage in consultations and diagnostic procedures, see patients in an office setting, and perform operations. In addition, depending on the practice setting, they teach residents, attend committee meetings, engage in research, and do paper work. All report that they spend time reading journals, an activity which is not noted as uniformly by other surgical specialist respondents. Some indicate that they have special interest areas (e.g., vascular aspects of neurological surgery, pediatric neurosurgery), but most see a variety of problems in patients of all ages.

There is a significant amount of night and weekend call reported in this specialty, ranging from a solo practitioner on call "300 days a year" to every fourth night and weekend.

What Abilities and Talents Are Important in Neurological Surgery?

"It has been considered a cliche that manual dexterity is important. But in my own discipline of microvascular surgery I find that this is mandatory and, if anything, does not receive enough emphasis." The necessary talents and abilities in neurological surgery are summarized in this manner: "It takes an unusual combination of manual dexterity, patience, compulsion for detail, organizational skills, and a high confidence level . . ." to be a neurological surgeon.

What Personality Traits Best Characterize Neurological Surgeons?

Many phrases were used to describe neurological surgeons: "very exacting and perfectionistic"; "calm under pressure"; "strong, even domineering personalities"; "deliberate"; "inquisitive"; "direct"; to quote a few. Although one says, "there are no characteristics which can describe the great variability of physicians in neurosurgery," a pattern of an independent-minded individual with an interest in solving complex problems in an organized manner emerges.

What Advice Would You Give a Medical Student Interested in Neurological Surgery?

The time commitment necessary is emphasized by all respondents. "The time investment and level of commitment puts a strain on one's personal life, as well as one's family. Adequate support systems should be in place at home prior to consideration of this kind of training and subsequent career choice."

Advice is given concerning academic preparation: "Learn neuroanatomy and neurophysiology 'cold', be an excellent clinical neurologist, and do lab work in which you get to see an animal's brain."

Looking ahead to practice years, a warning is given, "the threat of malpractice action is a daily companion."

What Are the Future Challenges to Neurological Surgery?

Advances in technology are the dominant answers. One respondent adds another interesting aspect to the future of neurological surgery: "As the future of medicine progresses, preventive medicine assumes an important role. This will eventually impact on the neurological surgeon [who] must assume added responsibilities towards avoidance of disease rather than the crisis intervention we are practicing now. Major advances are yet to be seen with nervous system neoplasia, trauma, and congenital defects, the areas that will require the most thought and innovation from the new generation of neurological surgeons."

REFERENCES

1. Rovit RL, Weiss MH, Clark K. Letter to third-year medical students. American Association of Neurological Surgeons/ Congress of Neurological Surgery, Society of Neurological Surgeons. January 1984.
2. Physician characteristics and distribution in the United States, 2010. Chicago: American Medical Association, Table 6.4, p.441.
3. Leigh JP, Kravitz RL, Schembri M, Samuels SJ, Mobley S. Physician career satisfaction across specialties. *Arch Intern Med* 2002; 162:1577-1584.

Job Values Selection of Neurological Surgeons

You can complete the questionnaires and obtain your scores for all specialties online at http://www.sdn.net, or compare your job values (as recorded in the Appendix) with the job values of neurological surgeon respondents below:

Neurological Surgeons' Choices:	My Choices:
1. Creativity	1. _____
1. Independence	2. _____
1. Working with my hands	3. _____
1. Variety	4. _____
(there is a four-way tie for first place)	

No one chose: Sufficient time off

Summary Profile of Neurological Surgeons (derived from questionnaire answers)	My Personal Profile as a Neurological Surgeon				
They tend to:	I tend to: (circle one number)				
	Never	Rarely	Sometimes	Frequently	Always
Ask why	1	2	3	4	5
Pay attention to details	1	2	3	4	5
Enjoy taking care of people	1	2	3	4	5
Become bored with repetitive activity	1	2	3	4	5
Like complex problem solving	1	2	3	4	5
Value independence highly	1	2	3	4	5
Have manual dexterity	1	2	3	4	5
Need to see tangible results of their efforts quickly	1	2	3	4	5
Be energetic/have a high energy level	1	2	3	4	5
Be self-confident	1	2	3	4	5

Add total of numbers circled to get your TOTAL SCORE: _____

Transfer score to the Appendix.

Neurological surgery

sounds like me _____

could be a possibility _____

doesn't sound like me at all _____

Neurology

FAST FACTS:

Number of first year residency positions offered in 2011 : 266

Filled with US grads in 2011 : 59.8 %

Number of second year positions offered in 2011 : 339

Filled with US grads in 2011 : 60.8 %

Competitiveness: Moderate

Length of training: Adult neurology: 4 years (requires a preliminary year in general internal medicine with a minimum of eight months of internal medicine)

Number of residency programs offering first year positions: 60; offering second year positions: 75

Number of residents in training: 1,825

US senior matched applicants' mean Step 1 score: 225

US senior matched applicants' mean Step 2 score: 231

Number in US Board Certified in Neurology: 9,780

Staring median compensation: $220,000

Median compensation for all physicians in specialty: $250,000

Average work hours per week: 55

THE NEUROLOGIST IS CONCERNED WITH THE DIAGNOSIS AND treatment of disorders of the nervous system—the brain, spinal cord, and peripheral nerves, and certain muscle disorders and pain problems, especially headache. Many neurologic disorders require long-term care, and some are untreatable. There are close ties between the specialties of neurology and psychiatry—board certification is offered by a combined board of psychiatry and neurology—and practitioners often consult with each other on patient care.

Coombs' study[1] reports that medical students view the neurologist as being similar to the internist—"specialists in both fields seem to have similar kinds of logical, analytic minds and an academic orientation; and both types 'think a lot' and enjoy solving puzzles."

Residency Information. Both first and second year positions for adult neurology are offered through the NRMP Match. Competitive applicants have interest in clinical neuroscience and successfully complete a clinical or research neurology or neurosurgical elective.

In residency, you will receive training in both adult and child neurology and psychiatry. Those who are interested in specializing in child neurology must apply through the San Francisco Matching Program. Applicants need to successfully complete two years of training in pediatrics, or one year of pediatrics and a PG-1 year in neurology, or one year of pediatrics plus one year of basic neuroscience training. Training in child neurology itself is a three year program: one year in clinical adult neurology, one year "flexible" training, and one year in clinical child neurology. There were 80 residents in program year 1 of child neurology in 2009.

There are a small number of five year combined residency positions in internal medicine/neurology and psychiatry/neurology. There is also a seven year combined residency program in neurology/diagnostic radiology/neuroradiology. These programs participate in the NRMP.

After residency, many neurologists do fellowship training in a subspecialty area such as epilepsy (approved in December 2010), stroke, multiple sclerosis, and movement disorders. Fellowships are for one or two years.

Board Certification. After completing four years of training with at least three of the years in a neurology residency program, you may apply to the American Board of Psychiatry and Neurology to take Part

I of the certifying examination. This written examination includes questions on both neurology and psychiatry. Upon successful completion of Part I, you may apply for Part II, an oral examination.

The testing procedure for neurology with specialty qualifications in child neurology is the same as for neurology, except that in Part II there is more emphasis on child neurology than on clinical neurology. There is also a subspecialty certificate in clinical neurophysiology.

It is possible to seek certification in both psychiatry and neurology. You must complete six to seven years of postgraduate training with two to three years in each specialty plus a clinical first year. To achieve board certification in both child psychiatry and child neurology you must be certified in general psychiatry before applying for the examination in child psychiatry and meet the requirements for certification in neurology with special qualification in child neurology.

Supply and Projections. The number of self-designated neurologists has more than tripled from 5685 in 1980 to 15,212. [2] Of these, child neurologists number more than 1300. Advances in therapies, new diagnostic techniques and the aging population are thought to be factors that will increase demand for neurologists.

Economic Status and Types of Practice. Neurologists' compensation is reported to be a bit higher than the national average. Most are in clinical practices in metropolitan areas and some are becoming hospitalists. The most common area of clinical focus is headache, followed by epilepsy, stroke, and electroencephalography. [3]

Further Information. The American Academy of Neurology, 1080 Montreal Avenue, St. Paul, MN 55116. Telephone: (800) 879-1960. Internet address: www.aan.com. Free student membership. The website has a section dedicated to medical students including information about the specialty, frequently asked questions, training data, and how to form a Student Interest Group in Neurology (SIGN) at your school.

A COMPOSITE PICTURE OF THE NEUROLOGIST
Why Choose Neurology?

Intellectual challenge and the influence of a teacher were two factors that attracted the respondents to neurology. Neurologists say that they would not want to practice surgery or obstetrics which have "too many routine procedures" or pediatrics with its "excessive well-child care."

An intriguing survey, conducted among 576 male and female neurologists at a neurology conference, found that the rate of migraines among headache specialists is 60 to 70 percent, contrasted with about 10 percent in the general population. This led the survey authors to conclude that, "A personal history of migraine may stimulate an interest in neurology." [4]

What Do You Like Most About Neurology?

The variety and complexity of diseases is intellectually stimulating and most enjoyable to neurologists. One respondent says, "It's like being a detective." The number of "very satisfied" neurologists (39%) is slightly lower than the total sample (42.3 percent) , but those "dissatisfied" (16.2 percent) is also lower than the national sample (17.6 percent). [5]

What Do You Like Least About Neurology?

A diversity of factors cause frustration: emergency care, patients with problems that have no effective treatment, and the need to perform "unnecessary and complete neurologic evaluations when the diagnosis is already obvious."

What Is Your Typical Daily Schedule?

Neurologists who provide primary care for their patients, in addition to neurologic consultations, have practices that may resemble general internists' practices. One respondent limits his practice to neurology and says, "A typical day in my work is going to the hospital at 7:30 AM, rounding on one or two of my own patients, following up on three or four consultations, reviewing CT scans and x-rays on these patients, and discussing individual patients with other physicians either in the lounge or by phone. I usually reach my office around 9:00 AM and see patients through 4:00 PM. I see approximately 25 new patients a week. Most of them are referred by their primary care physicians. I also see approximately 40 return patients in a week. These patients are either followed for a short period of time until their immediate problem is resolved or I follow them for a long time caring for their chronic problems. I see the 'bread and butter' of neurology, that is, migraine and vertigo most often. However, I also see a whole spectrum of neurologic disorders and complaints ranging from sensory, motor, cerebellar, and cognitive disorders to primary muscle disease."

Child neurologists typically treat seizures, headache, hyperactivity, and developmental delay.

What Abilities and Talents Are Important in Neurology?

"Individuals who like to figure out problems and are mathematically and analytically oriented are best suited for neurology where the physical examination provides very concrete objective evidence that can be pieced together with the history to make a specific diagnosis."

"It is especially important to be able to listen to the patient's history—it can often be critical in making the diagnosis."

What Personality Traits Best Characterize Neurologists?

Neurologists have an image of being "brainy" and emotionally withdrawn from patients.[1] Respondents do see themselves as inquisitive and intellectual types. Other traits that characterize them are "perfectionistic," "intense," and "compulsive."

The Myers-Briggs Type Indicator data report that neurologists are similar in personality traits to neurosurgeons, but that neurology attracts more introverts and neurological surgery, more extroverts. Neurologists are thoughtful and scholarly and work in a specialty that requires understanding of complex problems in terms of cause-and-effect. Independent, academic types seem to be attracted to this field.

What Advice Would You Give a Medical Student Interested in Neurology?

"Choose a neurology residency that offers a wide spectrum of patients and pathology. This should include not only a large hospital with acutely ill neurologic patients, but also an out-patient facility for long-term, follow-up, and out-patient workup of neurologic problems which can be done at the residency level."

Another respondent says that medical students interested in child neurology should "learn about children with more subtle neurologic illnesses, e.g., learning disorders and behavior problems."

What Are the Future Challenges to Neurology?

Feinberg[6] suggests a reordering of priorities in the teaching of neurology, advocating emphasis on "chronic diseases or diseases curable in ambulatory care settings."

Practice innovations include telemedicine – consults via telephone, the Internet, and live video technology to rural areas. Technological advances have allowed new treatment capabilities for diseases such as multiple sclerosis, brain tumors and strokes.

A declining number of neurologists are entering research and the challenge exists to "combine the explosion of beneficial discoveries and findings of research in the neurosciences with clinical practice to benefit patients." The success of the Human Genome Project is predicted to "...revolutionize our appreciation of gene action in both neurological function and disease."[7]

REFERENCES

1. Coombs RH. *Mastering medicine.* New York: The Free Press, 1978, pp. 203–205.
2. Physician Characteristics and Distribution, 2010. American Medical Association. Table 6.2,   p. 439.
3. Swarztrauber K, Keran CM and the members of the AAN Practice Characteristics Subcommittee. Neurologists 1998. St. Paul, MN: American Academy of Neurology, Table 15, p. 10.
4. Carey B. How do doctors treat their own severe headaches? The Oregonian, March 16,2002, pp. L1 & 5.

5. Leigh JP, Kravitz RL, Schembri M, Samuels SJ, Mobley S. Physician career satisfaction across specialties. *Arch Intern Med* 2002; 162:1577-1584.
6. Feinberg DM. Correspondence. Redesigning graduate medical education—location and content. *N Engl J Med* 1996;335(19):1459.
7. Rosenberg RN. Genomics and the transformation of neurology. *JAMA* 2001;286(22):2869-2870.

Job Values Selection of Neurologists

You can complete the questionnaires and obtain your scores for all specialties online at http://www.sdn.net, or compare your job values (as recorded in the Appendix) with the job values of neurologist respondents below:

Neurologists' Choices:	My Choices:
1. Working with my mind	1. _____
1. Good income	2. _____
2. Creativity	3. _____
2. Independence	4. _____
2. Working with people	
(there are ties for first and second place)	

No one chose: Working with my hands, sufficient time off

Summary Profile of Neurologists **My Personal Profile as a Neurologist**
(derived from questionnaire answers)

They tend to:	I tend to: (circle one number)				
	Never	Rarely	Sometimes	Frequently	Always
Ask why	1	2	3	4	5
Become bored with repetitive activity	1	2	3	4	5
Like complex problem solving	1	2	3	4	5
Need control over a situation	1	2	3	4	5
Value independence highly	1	2	3	4	5
Prefer a planned schedule	1	2	3	4	5
Accept long term outcomes	1	2	3	4	5
Think logically	1	2	3	4	5
Be perfectionistic	1	2	3	4	5
Be scholarly	1	2	3	4	5

Add total of numbers circled to get your TOTAL SCORE:_____

Transfer score to the Appendix.

Neurology

sounds like me _____

could be a possibility _____

doesn't sound like me at all _____

Nuclear Medicine

FAST FACTS:

Total number of first year program positions to be offered in 2010: 107 (third year after graduation from medical school)

Length of training: 3 years (if preceded by one year of a transitional or preliminary program); 2 years (if preceded by completion of a residency in another specialty); 1 year (if preceded by completion of a diagnostic radiology program)

Number of residency programs: 55

Number of residents in training: 152

Competitiveness: Low

Number In US Board Certified In Nuclear Medicine: 505

Median compensation for early career: $286,000

Median compensation for all physicians in specialty: $317,000

Average work hours per week: 48

AS NEW RADIOLOGIC TECHNIQUES RAPIDLY WERE DEVELOPED in the 1960s there was active interest in nuclear medicine, not just by radiologists but also by physicians in other specialties. A conjoint board composed of representatives of the American Board of Internal Medicine, the American Board of Pathology, the American Board of Radiology, and the Society of Nuclear Medicine was established in 1971.

Nuclear medicine is defined as ". . . the medical specialty that uses small amounts of radioactive materials for diagnosis, and somewhat larger amounts for treatment of diseases."[1] It differs from x-rays or from computed tomography (CT) scans in that the radiation source is not a machine passing radiation through a patient's body but is inside the patient for a brief time and is detected by special equipment. In nuclear medicine, greater emphasis is placed on the function of an organ rather than the structure of the organ as in radiology. There are two types of nuclear medicine tests: in vitro (in the test tube) procedures, analyzing blood and urine specimens using radiochemicals; and in vivo (in the body) procedures, evaluating organ function or appearance after the patient has been given small amounts of radiopharmaceuticals.

Residency Information. Residencies in this specialty were first offered in 1975. The two years of training in nuclear medicine usually are preceded by two years of internal medicine, pathology, or radiology. This is becoming extremely rare as a way to train in nuc med. The vast majority of trainees in nuc med are either radiology trained or using it as a springboard to a radiology residency.

Board Certification. Following successful completion of two years of a clinical postdoctoral residency and two years of a nuclear medicine residency, you may apply to take the written certifying examination.

Supply and Projections. Technological advances may determine the job market in this field.

Economic Status and Types of Practice. Nuclear medicine earn above average incomes. It is becoming more difficult to get a job as a non-radiology trained nuc med physician as hospitals and groups want people who can read both nuclear studies and other imaging modalities.

Further Information. The Society of Nuclear Medicine, 1850 Samuel Morse Drive, Reston, VA 20190. Telephone: (703) 326-1190. Internet address: www.snm.org.

A COMPOSITE PICTURE OF THE NUCLEAR MEDICINE PHYSICIAN

Respondents are all in full-time practice of nuclear medicine. Some are board certified in both internal medicine and nuclear medicine; others are board certified in radiology and nuclear medicine.

Why Choose Nuclear Medicine?

Almost all respondents were attracted to nuclear medicine as a new field with a technological orientation: "There are lots of possibilities for innovation, experimentation, and creativity." It was seen as an area of medicine that would be "always changing with the advances in technology."

In addition, it offered predictable work hours, good income, and job opportunities. Respondents' reactions to other specialties included: that they would not want to practice emergency medicine, "too stressful"; radiology or pathology, "too little patient contact"; a primary care specialty, "extremely difficult to keep abreast of all areas equally well"; and surgery, "I am the wrong personality type." One respondent sums up the appeal of nuclear medicine: "I was attracted by the mix of problems encountered in nuclear medicine, the less direct patient care for trivial problems, and the good salaries."

What Do You Like Most About Nuclear Medicine?

The variety and creative process is most enjoyable to respondents: "Every day brings new questions, new concepts, and new information." Because findings are "more reliable than other aspects of medicine" there is the "satisfaction of helping other physicians solve tough clinical problems." Many respondents enjoy the opportunities to do research.

What Do You Like Least About Nuclear Medicine?

Most frustrations relate to administrative tasks and complying with regulatory agencies. Also, nuclear medicine physicians do not like "being treated as technicians and not consulted about specific cases" and "indefinite test results."

What Is Your Typical Daily Schedule?

The day is generally divided into clinical, administrative, teaching, and research activities. The work includes supervising both diagnostic and laboratory procedures, as well as interpreting those procedures. Respondents report an average day of from 8 to 10 hours; nuclear medicine physicians rarely are required to return to the hospital after regular work hours. Even those in private practice are engaged in research, writing reports, and preparing conferences, unlike other medical specialties where much of this type of activity is centered in the academic centers. The small numbers of full-time nuclear medicine physicians and the rapidly evolving data base and technology have resulted in this type of work schedule.

What Abilities and Talents Are Important in Nuclear Medicine?

Interest in instrumentation and computers and a good foundation in physical sciences are important in nuclear medicine. You also need to be visually oriented in order to interpret scan data.

What Personality Traits Characterize Nuclear Medicine Physicians?

"Curious," "innovative," and "low key" are the most commonly reported traits. Respondents see themselves as "willing to accommodate to advances in technology," which often means learning new things constantly. The Myers-Briggs Type Indicator data indicate that nuclear medicine attracts physicians who "like to be in the very forefront of knowledge where applications can be made to real problems."

What Advice Would You Give a Medical Student Interested in Nuclear Medicine?

Most respondents advise to "get a solid background in medicine and radiology. Do not underestimate the value of clinical acumen and judgment." However, if you are clinically oriented, one respondent recommends radiology rather than nuclear medicine. (Ed. note: It's all a matter of opinion, again. Most physicians in clinical specialties would not view radiology as a "clinically oriented specialty.")

An interest in research and some expertise in computers and statistics are recommended. Graduate training should provide exposure to all imaging modalities, not just nuclear medicine procedures; some people recommend taking primary board certification in medicine or radiology in addition to nuclear medicine.

What Are the Future Challenges to Nuclear Medicine?

Continued growth in the face of government cost containment is a recurrent theme: "Government payment plans may make acquisition of expensive hospital equipment more difficult, as well as discourage its use for radiology/nuclear medicine procedures." Also challenging is the need to ". . . correlate nuclear techniques with more automated imaging modalities to define the most effective, least expensive, safest techniques for a specific diagnostic problem."

REFERENCE

1. American College of Nuclear Physicians. *What is nuclear medicine?* Washington, DC: American College of Nuclear Physicians.

Job Values Selection of Nuclear Medicine Physicians

You can complete the questionnaires and obtain your scores for all specialties online at http://www.sdn.net, or compare your job values (as recorded in the Appendix) with the job values of nuclear medicine respondents below:

Nuclear Medicine Physicians' Choices:	My Choices:
1. Creativity	1. _____
2. Independence	2. _____
2. Good income	3. _____
2. Achievement	4. _____
2. Variety	
(there is a four-way tie for second place)	

No one chose: Working with my hands, taking care of patients, feedback from others.

Summary Profile of Nuclear Medicine Physicians
(derived from questionnaire answers)

My Personal Profile as a Nuclear Medicine Physician

They tend to:	I tend to: (circle one number)				
	Never	Rarely	Sometimes	Frequently	Always
Ask why	1	2	3	4	5
Pay attention to details	1	2	3	4	5
Need to see tangible results of their efforts quickly	1	2	3	4	5
Accept schedule disruptions	1	2	3	4	5
Be uncomfortable with poorly defined problems	1	2	3	4	5
Like gadgets and enjoy technology	1	2	3	4	5
Be scholarly	1	2	3	4	5
Adapt to changes easily	1	2	3	4	5
Be mathematically inclined	1	2	3	4	5
Be visually oriented	1	2	3	4	5

Add total of numbers circled to get your TOTAL SCORE:_____

Transfer score to the Appendix.

Nuclear medicine

sounds like me _____

could be a possibility _____

doesn't sound like me at all _____

Obstetrics and Gynecology

TWO SEPARATE FIELDS, OBSTETRICS AND GYNECOLOGY, ARE combined to provide health care to women. The obstetrician cares for the woman before, during, and after her pregnancy; the gynecologist cares for disorders and diseases of the female reproductive tract. You may combine both areas in your practice or you may concentrate on one; your training will encompass both obstetrics and gynecology.

In the past, medical students may have had a poorly defined image of this specialty, with Coombs[1] reporting nearly 40 percent of freshmen students having "no opinion" about obstetrics and gynecology. He attributes this to the fact that a majority of medical students were male and, therefore, did not have personal experience with this field. Today, perhaps reflecting the increased percentage of female medical students, 79.7% of the residents in this specialty are female. [2]

Residency Information. Reflecting the new emphasis on primary care in obstetrics and gynecology, there is a mandatory minimum of six months of primary care training in the four-year program.

Board Certification. A written examination may be taken upon the successful completion of four years of residency training. Those who pass need to engage in two years of practice prior to taking the oral examination. Those who enter a two-year postresidency fellowship need six months of practice experience prior to the oral examination.

Certificates of special competence are awarded in maternal-fetal medicine, critical care medicine, gynecologic oncology, hospice and palliative medicine, and reproductive endocrinology/infertility.

Supply and Projections. Rayburn[3] has issued a new workforce report projecting that there will be a shortage of obstetricians and gynecologists. The US population of women is expected to grow 43% from 2010 to 2050 and the average age of women will be higher. A factor contributing to the possible shortage are the changes in work priorities with the average age for a female obstetrician to stop practicing obstetrics at 43 years and a male obstetrician at 49 years. In addition, there is a severe geographic maldistribution with many rural counties having less than one ob-gyn per 10,000 women.

Economic Status and Types of Practice. Obstetricians-gynecologists have high incomes but they are below the median earnings of their surgical colleagues. Contributing to their inequity with subspecialty surgical specialists are higher malpractice liability premiums and office personnel salaries.

The majority are in private fee-for-service practice with a trend toward group practice. There is a rapidly growing hospitalist/laborist model of care that is attracting younger physicians in this specialty. [4] Those who have finished fellowships in subspecialties of obstetrics and gynecology often practice in an academic environment, doing research, teaching, and patient care. There are also career opportunities in public health: as planners, consultants, and administrators in maternal and child health and family planning agencies at local, national, or international levels.

Further Information. The American College of Obstetrics and Gynecology, 409 12th Street SW, Washington, DC 20024. Telephone: (202) 638-5577. Internet address: www.acog.org.

A video to introduce medical students to this specialty has been produced and distributed to medical schools. There is information for students on the website about guidelines for applying to residencies in obstetrics and gynecology.

The American College of Osteopathic Obstetricians and Gynecologists, 409 12th Street, SW, P.O. Box 96920, Washington, D.C. 20090.

A COMPOSITE PICTURE OF AN OBSTETRICIAN-GYNECOLOGIST

Why Choose Obstetrics and Gynecology?

The appeal of obstetrics and gynecology was remarkably similar among the respondents as they all stressed its multidisciplinary nature: "It combines medical and surgical treatment modalities in situations where patients can usually be helped." "A wide variety of interests may be stimulated through this field. It is a combination of medicine, surgery, primary care, and emergency medicine."

One respondent says, "I thought of being an internist, but there wasn't any surgery; I thought of being a surgeon, but there wasn't any internal medicine." Family medicine is considered to be "too broad"; whereas, psychiatry, ophthalmology, and dermatology are "too narrow." Internal medicine has "too many chronic problems" and pathology and radiology lack sufficient patient contact.

What Do You Like Most About Obstetrics and Gynecology?

Even though physicians who were surveyed are attracted by the multidisciplinary aspects, most like the surgery best. Of specific value are "curing problems," "good outcomes," and "diagnosing and managing high-risk obstetric complications antepartum and subsequently bringing the patient and fetus to a successful outcome." Some attain a high degree of satisfaction from ". . . the close interpersonal relationship that frequently develops between the patient and her physician," "the joy of participating in childbirth," and "the opportunity to help couples who are suffering from infertility establish a pregnancy." A statistically significant percentage of physicians in this specialty report that they are "dissatisfied" (24.2 percent) with only 34.4 percent, "very satisfied." This is possibly due to high medical legal risks and high expectations for good birth outcomes.[5]

What Do You Like Least About Obstetrics and Gynecology?

Respondents confirm the image of this specialty as involving long hours and an irregular schedule. "Night call and interruption of (my) daily schedule by obstetrical patients in labor" and "the time infringement on my family and personal life" are cited as the least liked aspects of their specialty. Also disliked is "the present day medicolegal environment which makes obstetrics and gynecology a 'high risk' specialty."

What Is Your Typical Daily Schedule?

"It is hard to say what 'typical' is—I'm not sure there is such a thing. Today I went to the hospital at 2:00 AM to deliver a baby; got to bed at 4:30 AM; up at 8:00 AM to go to the hospital and make rounds; had another delivery at 10:00 AM; got to the office at 10:40 AM (40 minutes late for office patients); at 12:30 PM, back to the hospital to do a tubal ligation; 2:00 PM, back in the office; at 5:00 PM went to a hospital committee meeting; home at 8:00 PM."

Respondents report that they spend a few half-days per week in surgery and the rest of the time in the office. They work from 10 to 12 hours a day and frequently do their own deliveries even if they are not "on call." Most patients are healthy young women who come for prenatal care or medical examinations.

What Abilities and Talents Are Important in Obstetrics and Gynecology?

Although obstetrics and gynecology is a surgical specialty, the level of manual dexterity does not need to be as delicate as for the ophthalmologist or neurosurgeon: "Surgical skills are required, but most can be learned."

What is needed is "an ability to listen and empathize with women's problems." In addition, you need to have the dedication and willingness to put in long hours and to tolerate an irregular schedule.

What Personality Traits Best Characterize Obstetricians-Gynecologists?

Although obstetricians-gynecologists described themselves as "generally calm in tense situations," they also view themselves as "energetic," "outgoing," and "animated." An explanation for this apparent contradiction may be that they describe themselves as "sensitive to the emotional, psychosocial, and physical needs of their patients" but are easily adaptable to changing conditions.

In the Myers-Briggs Type Indicator studies, obstetrician-gynecologists are reported to be similar to orthopaedic surgeons in personality, both liking discrete problems that have concrete, immediate solutions in contrast to problems that deal with chronic care or psychiatry. McCaulley[6] observes, "Obstetrics and gynecology is a fascinating specialty from the point of view of psychological type theory, because its tasks call on opposing processes which are unlikely to be highly developed in the same person."

The nature of this specialty seems to require a temperament that can be comfortable in offering psychological support and managing a case by "waiting," as well as performing highly technical surgical skills, sometimes in a crisis situation. In the past, many obstetricians and gynecologists have been technically oriented and, therefore, have been judged to be authoritarian in patient care and less sensitive to psychological issues. The pressure from patients for more compassion may attract physicians who are more psychologically oriented in temperament.

What Advice Would You Give a Medical Student Interested in Obstetrics and Gynecology?

The advice is not encouraging: "Be prepared to be up at night more than any other specialty and be prepared to be sued for malpractice more than any other specialty." "Choose obstetrics-gynecology only if you are willing to work hard, day or night and are willing to accept the major role the patient or family has in most obstetrics-gynecology decisions."

Most residency programs consider away electives beneficial because being known in a program may improve an applicant's odds of matching.[7]

What Are the Future Challenges to Obstetrics and Gynecology?

The overwhelming challenge is related to social and economic issues—competition from family physicians, general internists, midwives, naturopaths, and chiropractors; the legal, ethical, and moral issues concerning childbirth; and the malpractice crisis, i.e., "combating nuisance lawsuits and excessive settlements so that there is less defensive medicine and more humane, noninterventionist practice."

Future challenges within the field also involve the development and refinement of new techniques, such as in vitro fertilization, embryo transplants, and the treatment of gynecologic malignancies.

REFERENCES

1. Coombs RH. *Mastering medicine.* New York: The Free Press, 1978, p. 193.
2. Brotherton SE, Etzel, SI. Graduate Medical Education, 2009-2010. JAMA 2010; 304(11):1256.

3. Rayburn WF. The Obsterician-Gynecologist Workforce in the US, Facts and Figures with Key Findings 2011. American College of Obstetrics and Gynecology. Reported in Lorenz RP, Chair's Report: A projection of an Ob-Gyn Shortage. www.acog.org accessed January 15, 2011.

4. Funk C, Anderson BL, Schulkin J, Weinstein L. Survey of obstetric and gynecologic hospitalists and laborists. *Am J Obstet Gynecol*, 2010Aug;203(2):177.e1-4.

5. Leigh JP, Kravitz RL, Schembri M, Samuels SJ,, Mobley S. Physician career satisfaction across specialties. *Arch Intern Med* 2002; 162:1577-1584.

6. McCaulley MH. Application of the Myers-Briggs Type Indicator to medicine and other health professions, Monograph I. Gainesville, FL: Center for Applications of Psychological Type, Inc., 1978, p. 241.

7. Metheny WP et al. Answers to applicant selection from a directory of residency programs in obstetrics and gynecology. *Obstet & Gyn* 1996;88:133–136.

Job Values Selection of Obstetricians and Gynecologists

You can complete the questionnaires and obtain your scores for all specialties online at http://www.sdn.net, or compare your job values (as recorded in the Appendix) with the job values of obstetrician-gynecologist respondents below:

Obstetrician-Gynecologists' Choices:	My Choices:
1. Working with people	1. _____
1. Taking care of people	2. _____
1. Variety	3. _____
1. Working with my hands	4. _____
(there is a four-way tie for first place)	

No one chose: Prestige, feedback from others

Summary Profile of Obstetrician-Gynecologists (derived from questionnaire answers)	**My Personal Profile as an Obstetrician-Gynecologist**				
They tend to:	I tend to: (circle one number)				
	Never	Rarely	Sometimes	Frequently	Always
Enjoy taking care of people	1	2	3	4	5
Need to see tangible results of their efforts quickly	1	2	3	4	5
Be energized by people	1	2	3	4	5
Act decisively	1	2	3	4	5
Accept schedule disruptis	1	2	3	4	5
Think logically	1	2	3	4	5
Be objective	1	2	3	4	5
Be "doers" rather than talkers	1	2	3	4	5
Adapt to changes easily	1	2	3	4	5
Be calm in a crisis	1	2	3	4	5

Add total of numbers circled to get your TOTAL SCORE:_____

Transfer score to the Appendix.

Obstetrics and Gynecology

    sounds like me_____

    could be a possibility_____

    doesn't sound like me at all_____

Ophthalmology

ALTHOUGH OPHTHALMOLOGY IS CLASSIFIED AS A SURGICAL specialty, ophthalmologists spend less time in the operating room than most surgeons. Many physicians find the mixture of medicine and surgery—"ranging from the prescription of lenses and standard medical treatment to the most delicate and precise surgical manipulations"—very appealing.[1]

Ophthalmology is concerned with the structure, function, diseases, and abnormalities of the eye. Patients of all ages, from newborn to geriatric, may seek ophthalmologic care: "newborns and infants with congenital defects; preschool children with strabismus; teenagers in need of glasses or contact lenses; adults with refraction problems, glaucoma, and injuries as well as patients with cataracts and retinal diseases."[2] Physicians more oriented toward surgery can be primarily involved in vitreoretinal surgery, glaucoma surgery, oculoplastic surgery, corneal transplantation, or other anterior segment microsurgery. The ophthalmologist can also have a more medically oriented practice, for example, in the field of neuro-ophthalmology or medical retinal disease management.

Residency Information. Ophthalmology is an "early match" specialty with results announced in January through the San Francisco Matching Program. Interviews are scheduled between October through December in a student's fourth year. You will be matched for a second year post-graduate position starting 18 months after the match. You will need to apply through the National Residency Matching Program (NRMP) for a first year post-graduate transitional training position.

There is an increasing trend to subspecialize in this specialty with one respondent estimating that 50 percent of residents do so.

Board Certification. You may take the written exam after completing your residency and, if you pass, must take the oral exam within two years. There are no board-certified subspecialties in ophthalmology, but fellowships are offered for those who wish further training in the subspecialty areas, such as cornea, glaucoma, neuro-ophthalmology, pediatric ophthalmology, and retina-vitreous.

Supply and Projections. With an increasing number of services provided by optometrists, this specialty may be oversupplied in some areas of the country.

Economic Status and Types of Practice. Most ophthalmologists are engaged in private fee-for-service practices in urban areas. Solo practice is popular because there are relatively few after-hours or weekend emergency calls. The income is lower than other subspecialty surgeons. Equipment costs for ophthalmologists are higher than for most other primarily office-based practices and many ophthalmologists employ at least two full-time assistants.

Further Information. The American Academy of Ophthalmology, 655 Beach Street, San Francisco, CA 94109. Telephone: (415) 561-8581. Internet address: www.aao.org

Information about the specialty, selecting and applying to a residency program and information about subspecialties is available through the link Young Ophthalmologists on the AAO website.

A COMPOSITE PICTURE OF THE OPHTHALMOLOGIST

Why Choose Ophthalmology?

Ophthalmology attracts individuals while they are in medical school: "I liked the relaxed attitude of the instructors in this specialty." Students also perceive this specialty as offering more variety and continuity than others: "As a student I saw that ophthalmology involved the complete care of patients; I could make the diagnosis, then treat, either medically or surgically."

Respondents who considered other surgical specialties as a career choice dismissed them on the basis of irregular hours (obstetrics-gynecology), too mechanical (urology), or too broad a field (general surgery). Ophthalmologists report that they are not attracted to psychiatry—"it is difficult to gauge the results of your efforts," or pediatrics—"too much hassle," "dealing only with children," and "long hours."

What Do You Like Most About Ophthalmology?

Ophthalmologists derive much pleasure from helping others: "It is most enjoyable to see a patient regain lost vision through some treatment I have rendered. The feeling of having done something worthwhile for that patient, something that improves the quality of his or her life, is the thing I enjoy most about my work."

Almost all the respondents cite "surgery," especially the challenge of microscopic techniques, as a positive factor in the specialty.

A statistically significant percentage of physicians in this specialty report that they are "dissatisfied" (21 percent) with 41.4 percent indicating "very satisfied." [3]

What Do You Like Least About Ophthalmology?

"Office routine" is the unanimous answer. Examples include "refractions (fitting for glasses)," "patients with minor problems and routine refractions can become monotonous," and "the boredom burnout that sometimes occurs with repetitive days in the office."

What Is Your Typical Daily Schedule?

The ophthalmologist's work week is approximately 50 hours long, 80 to 90 percent of which is spent in office practice. On a typical day, appointments are scheduled from 8:30 AM until 5:00 PM (with a short lunch break). Much time is spent doing routine eye examinations and refractions. In addition, there may be some emergencies (foreign objects in the eye, acute infections, or injuries). All surgery may be scheduled for one day, or a few hours on certain days. Surgical patients are usually followed postoperatively in the office for an extended period. Depending on the type of practice, the ophthalmologist may rotate hospital rounds with others or schedule them prior to office hours.

On-call schedules are lighter than other specialties. Many ophthalmologists volunteer their time in community preventive programs, such as glaucoma screening and eye bank associations.

What Abilities and Talents Are Important in Ophthalmology?

As in other surgical specialties, manual dexterity is imperative: "A considerable amount of dexterity and eye-hand coordination is needed to perform the microscopic surgery. Binocular vision and normal color vision are important." In addition, "surgical decisions require a calm, level-headed approach."

What Personality Traits Best Characterize Ophthalmologists?

Ophthalmologists see themselves as "compulsive," "perfectionistic," "even-tempered," and "detail-oriented." Patience is an important quality in both the nature of the work and in dealing with patients.

What Advice Would You Give a Medical Student Interested in Ophthalmology?

The message is clear: There are more applicants for residency positions than there are openings. "Competition is keen for residency positions. It would be best to spend a considerable amount of elective time in ophthalmology to be certain of one's interest, as well as demonstrating this to the program to which one might apply. It is beneficial to have done research or have authored publications."

However, some respondents issue a warning: "I would advise a medical student interested in ophthalmology to consider the possibility of another specialty because the field of ophthalmology has become extremely crowded and I find that younger ophthalmologists are resorting to many 'gimmicks' in order to build their practices."

What Are the Future Challenges to Ophthalmology?

"Increasing intrusion by nonmedical personnel" and "advances in surgery" are the answers given by all respondents.

The distinction between the ophthalmologist and the optometrist is often not well understood by the lay public and the optometrists are trying to expand their activities through legislation.

In addition to technological advances in surgery, there may be greater demands for surgical interventions because the American population base is aging, resulting in a higher incidence of degenerative eye diseases, cataracts, and glaucoma.

REFERENCES

1. American Academy of Ophthalmology, Association of University Professors of Ophthalmology. *Envision Ophthalmology.* San Francisco, American Academy of Ophthalmology, 1982.

2. Kalina RE. Letter. Seattle: Association of University Professors of Ophthalmology, 1983.

3. Leigh JP, Kravitz RL, Schembri M, Samuels SJ,, Mobley S. Physician career satisfaction across specialties. *Arch Intern Med* 2002; 162:1577-1584.

Job Values Selection of Ophthalmologists

You can complete the questionnaires and obtain your scores for all specialties online at http://www.sdn.net, or compare your job values (as recorded in the Appendix) with the job values of ophthalmologist respondents below:

Ophthalmologists' Choices:	My Choices:
1. Working with my hands	1. _____
2. Taking care of people	2. _____
3. Achievement	3. _____
4. Good income	4. _____
4. Independence	
(there is a tie for fourth place)	

No one chose: Creativity, decision making, feedback from others

Summary Profile of Ophthalmologists (derived from questionnaire answers)	My Personal Profile as an Ophthalmologist				

They tend to:	I tend to: (circle one number)				
	Never	Rarely	Sometimes	Frequently	Always
Pay attention to details	1	2	3	4	5
Enjoy taking care of people	1	2	3	4	5
Become bored with repetitive activity	1	2	3	4	5
Value time off	1	2	3	4	5
Have manual dexterity	1	2	3	4	5
Need to see tangible results of their efforts quickly	1	2	3	4	5
Prefer a planned schedule	1	2	3	4	5
Be achievers	1	2	3	4	5
Be perfectionistic	1	2	3	4	5
Be warm and sympathetic	1	2	3	4	5

Add total of numbers circled to get your TOTAL SCORE: _____

Transfer score to the Appendix.

Ophthalmology

sounds like me_____

could be a possibility_____

doesn't sound like me at all_____

Orthopaedic Surgery

THE "CELEBRITY" ATMOSPHERE IN SPORTS HAS BROUGHT much media attention to the medical specialty of orthopaedic surgery. Many orthopaedic surgeons are athletically inclined; it may be an interest in sports that initially attracts medical students to the specialty. However, orthopaedic surgery encompasses much more than trauma from sport-related injuries. Physicians in this specialty seek to restore normal function to a deformed, diseased, or injured part of the musculoskeletal system utilizing medical, surgical, and physical rehabilitation methods. There may be, in many cases, as much effort expended in the postoperative recovery period as in the initial time of treatment.

Residency Information. As in other surgical specialties, residency training is lengthy. The first year or two may be spent in a general surgery or other approved medical or surgical residency. The last three years must be taken in an orthopaedic surgery residency. Competitive applicants have high grades, a demonstrated interest in orthopaedics, and good motor skills.

Unlike ophthalmology and urology there are a relatively large number of first-year positions offered through the National Resident Matching Program. However, not all programs have arranged for a first-year of training. You will, therefore, need to apply to programs inside and outside the Match and to first-year (transitional) surgical programs. There are subspecialty training programs in adult reconstructive orthopaedics, foot and ankle surgery, hand surgery, musculoskeletal oncology, orthopaedic sports medicine, orthopaedic trauma, pediatric orthopaedics, reconstructive orthopaedics, and surgery of the spine for those already in an orthopaedic residency.

There are approximately 85 entry-level positions in osteopathic residencies.

Board Certification. After successful completion of your residency and two years in the clinical practice of orthopaedic surgery with at least 12 months in one location, you may apply to take the written examination for certification. Of the numerous subspecialty areas, only hand surgery and orthopaedic sports medicine offer separate certification.

Supply and Projections. The number of orthopaedic surgeons has doubled in the past 35 years. However, recent growth has been much slower.

Economic Status and Types of Practice. Orthopaedic surgeons' incomes are in the highest ranges of surgical subspecialists. However, professional liability insurance premiums are more expensive than those of many other specialists. Orthopaedic surgeons' offices often maintain expensive x-ray equipment and may employ a physical therapist.

A large percentage of orthopaedic physicians are in private fee-for-service practice, either solo or group. Generally, it is necessary to be in a medium- to large-size community to adequately support the practice.

Further Information. The American Academy of Orthopaedic Surgeons, 6300 N. River Road, Rosemont, IL 60018. Telephone: (847) 823-7186. Internet address: www.aaos.org.

A Postgraduate Orthopaedic Fellowships guide is published annually by the Academy.

A COMPOSITE PICTURE OF THE ORTHOPAEDIC SURGEON

Why Choose Orthopaedic Surgery?

Actual experiences in orthopaedic surgery made a strong impression on the respondents: "Involvement in the care of U.S. Army personnel, particularly those returning from the Viet Nam War during my period of serving as a surgeon assigned to the orthopaedic surgical service influenced my choice of specialty"; "I had a very positive rotation on orthopaedic surgery while a general surgery resident"; and "during my junior year I was assisting with the cast of a boy who had a fractured tibia. As I was watching the orthopaedic surgeons put the youngster's leg back together using hammers and screws and saws, I said to myself that this is what I want to do."

Some were initially interested in other specialties—"I enjoyed urology, but basically liked the younger folks in orthopaedics"; "there wasn't enough personal contact in anesthesia"; "there were more than an adequate number of general surgeons to supply the needs of most population areas." Respondents specifically cited internal medicine as a field they would not want to practice: "too cerebral," "too passive," "dealing with chronically ill patients who never really improve," "no immediate results." Respondents characterize obstetrics as having "too much repetition," "no real challenge," "only dealing with women."

What Do You Like Most About Orthopaedic Surgery?

Variety and challenge are the two aspects cited by all respondents. "It is variable from minute to minute, day to day, and has new things with new ways to approach them." "The ability to treat with one's hands and see immediate results" was considered an advantage.

A statistically significant percentage of physicians in this specialty report that they are "dissatisfied" (19.3 percent) with 47.1 percent indicating "very satisfied." This is a specialty where physicians were above the mean for both "very satisfied" and "dissatisfied," suggesting sharp differences of opinion.[1]

What Do You Like Least About Orthopaedic Surgery?

An unexpected aspect of the specialty for one respondent was "the amount of legal work we need to do." Dislike for this is expressed by respondents: "I spend a great deal of time testifying for lawyers and insurance companies in liability cases." Another finds "evaluating and treating Workers' Compensation and medical liability, back and neck pain problems," the least appealing part of his work. Others dislike "after-hours emergency room duty" and "people who are depressed and don't have the will to get well."

What Is Your Typical Daily Schedule?

Orthopaedic surgeons report working longer hours than most other physicians, several saying from 12 to 15 hours daily. A schedule might include early hospital rounds and surgery, emergency room visits, and office activities. In the office, time is spent not only in seeing patients but also in completing the heavy load of paperwork related to insurance forms and legal reports.

The patient population, a mixture of all ages, comes to the physician for a specific problem related to some part of their musculoskeletal system, but are otherwise generally in good health. Most patients will come to an orthopaedic surgeon only once in their lives, so each day will bring in "new" people and problems.

When "on call," orthopaedic surgeons are busy, "treating such things as a broken wrist, evaluating and setting up for surgery of a broken hip, or evaluating and putting on the operating room schedule a hand injury." There is a responsibility for emergency room coverage since major trauma cases often require the services of an orthopaedic surgeon.

What Abilities and Talents Are Important in Orthopaedic Surgery?

"Good hand coordination" and "a biomechanical mind" are necessary qualities. One respondent answers, "Some basic understanding of mechanics in regards to application of traction, application of varying fixation devices to bones, and in regards to function of specially organized body areas such as the flexor and extensor tendon system of the hand. Additionally, some reasonable proficiency with the orthopaedist's hands must be present, particularly to work under the microscope as in hand reconstruction surgery."

Also, "the everyday practice of orthopaedic surgery deals a great deal with pain problems and thus the orthopaedist does, I believe, need to have some ability to listen to patients with their problems and accept the fact that he [or she] is a 'pain oriented' physician."

What Personality Traits Best Characterize Orthopaedic Surgeons?

Orthopaedic surgeons describe themselves as "having a bias for action," "tending to be more objective and thinking in 'black and white' terms," and "liking to see results fast." However, one respondent warns that orthopaedists need to cultivate the patience to "look into the rather distant future—that is, weeks to months down the road, in regards to the results of treatment"—a task that may be difficult for some. The attraction in orthopaedic surgery is usually its action orientation, but the personality types most suited to this aspect do not find it as easy to deal with long-term problems or talking with patients.

What Advice Would You Give a Medical Student Interested in Orthopaedic Surgery?

"Decide early—it is extremely competitive." This is one of the specialties in which residency programs look favorably upon a clerkship during medical school as an evaluative method of choosing residents. It is, therefore, to your advantage (and may be even imperative in some programs) to take a clerkship in the residency program of your choice either in your third year or early in your fourth year.

Respondents advise students to "be sure you understand the emergency call at night and the long and arduous training period." They say "practice with a partner or two so that time off will be possible." Unlike some other specialties, problems cannot be put off until a later time; hence time commitment should be a major factor in evaluating the choice of an orthopaedic surgery specialty.

What Are the Future Challenges to Orthopaedic Surgery?

Scientific challenges include "improved operative techniques for joint replacements at areas other than the hips and knees, research combined between orthopaedic surgery and internal medicine in regards to osteoporosis, and continued advancements in regards to microsurgery. . . ."

Other challenges, not as positive, are the "fragmentation by the diffuse fields covered by orthopaedics" and "increasing malpractice litigation."

REFERENCE

1. Leigh JP, Kravitz RL, Schembri M, Samuels SJ,, Mobley S. Physician career satisfaction across specialties. *Arch Intern Med* 2002; 162:1577-1584.

Job Values Selection of Orthopaedic Surgeons

You can complete the questionnaires and obtain your scores for all specialties online at http://www.sdn.net, or compare your job values (as recorded in the Appendix) with the job values of orthopaedic surgeons:

Orthopaedic Surgeons' Choices:	My Choices:
1. Creativity	1. _____
1. Independence	2. _____
1. Decision making	3. _____
1. Taking care of people	4. _____
(there is a four-way tie for first place)	

No one chose: Good income, security, prestige, achievement, sufficient time off, or feedback from others

Summary Profile of Orthopaedic Surgeons (derived from questionnaire answers)	My Personal Profile as an Orthopaedic Surgeon				
They tend to:	I tend to: (circle one number)				
	Never	Rarely	Sometimes	Frequently	Always
Enjoy taking care of people	1	2	3	4	5
Become bored with repetitive activity	1	2	3	4	5
Value independence highly	1	2	3	4	5
Have manual dexterity	1	2	3	4	5
Need to see tangible results of their efforts quickly	1	2	3	4	5
Be energized by people	1	2	3	4	5
Act decisively	1	2	3	4	5
Be adventurous/like challenges	1	2	3	4	5
Be willing to work long hours	1	2	3	4	5
Be "doers" rather than talkers	1	2	3	4	5

Add total of numbers circled to get your TOTAL SCORE:_____

Transfer score to the Appendix.

Orthopaedic surgery

sounds like me _____

could be a possibility _____

doesn't sound like me at all _____

Otolaryngology – Head and Neck Surgery

FAST FACTS:

Number of first year residency positions offered in the NRMP in 2011 : 283

Filled with US grads in 2011 : 95.1%

Length of training: 5-6 years, including a PGY-1 year with at least 9 months of basic surgical, emergency and critical care and anesthesia training.

Number of residency programs: 105

Number of residents in training: 1,406

Competitiveness Rank: Highly competitive

Selection criteria for interview/ranking: good performance at elective at residency program, letters of recommendation from otolaryngologists, AOA membership, USMLE step 1 score, research experience and publication.

US senior matched applicants' mean Step 1 score: 240

US senior matched applicants' mean Step 2 score: 246

Number in US Board Certified in specialty: 8,035

Starting median compensation: $250,000

Median compensation for all physicians in specialty: $425,000

Average work hours per week: 54

THE EARLIEST SPECIALIZATION IN MEDICINE INVOLVED THOSE physicians who treat the eye, ear, nose, and throat. The first specialty boards were created in ophthalmology (1916) and otolaryngology

(1924). Coombs[1] speculates that these two fields were able to specify the qualifications and training objectives earlier than other areas of medicine that deal with less well-defined problems and less specific areas of the body.

The word otolaryngology is derived from the Greek base words: *otos,* meaning ear; *rhis,* meaning nose; and *larynx,* meaning throat. However, modern otolaryngology is no longer confined to the areas of ear, nose, and throat. It has become a comprehensive discipline of medicine and surgery of the head and neck region and the otolaryngologist is defined as ". . . a regional surgeon dealing with virtually all diseases and lesions above the clavicle, except for visual and eye-related disorders (ophthalmology) and lesions of the brain (neurosurgery, neurology)."[2] In 1980, The American Academy of Otolaryngology approved a name change to "Otolaryngology–Head and Neck Surgery" to reflect the evolution of the specialty. Reference to physicians in this field as "ENT (ear, nose, throat) doctor" is strongly discouraged; "otolaryngologist" is acceptable, but "head and neck surgeon" is preferred.

A trend toward subspecialization is increasing. All residents have training in at least the seven recognized subdivisions: otology, rhinology, laryngology, allergy, head and neck surgery, facial plastic and reconstructive surgery, and bronchoesophagology. A one or two-year fellowship following residency is available in any of the above subspecialty areas as well as in otology-neurotology, pediatric otolaryngology, plastic surgery within the head and neck and sleep medicine.

Residency Information. Before entering an otolaryngology training program, you must complete one to two years of general surgery, which is then followed by four years of an otolaryngology residency.

Many programs have made arrangements for a first year for their matched residents, but some have not. Therefore, you will want to apply to a number of first-year surgical programs to ensure a first-year position.

Otolaryngology is a very competitive specialty. There may be as many as 50 to 70 applicants for the three to four first-year places in a residency program.

Board Certification. One year of general surgery and four years of otolaryngology residency are required prior to written and oral examinations.

Supply and Projections. In the past 20 years, the number of otolaryngologists has not increased as dramatically as the other surgical specialists and, therefore, there is a projected shortage in this specialty. Many practices are hiring nurse practitioners and physician assistants to work in a team-based approach to patient care. However, there is concern that more training is needed for the physician extenders. [3]

Economic Status and Types of Practice. Most otolaryngologists are in private practices. They have above average incomes.

Further Information. The American Academy of Otolaryngology–Head and Neck Surgery. 1650 Diagonal Road, Alexandria, VA 22314. Telephone: (703) 836-4444. Internet address: www.entnet.org.

Information on residency requirements, current residency and fellowships vacancies, a mailing list of training program directors, including the structure of their programs, and other helpful information is available through the Academy office listed above.

A COMPOSITE PICTURE OF THE OTOLARYNGOLOGIST

Why Choose Otolaryngology?

Most respondents were interns or residents in other specialties when they decided to switch to otolaryngology. "I liked internal medicine, but enjoyed the anatomy and challenge of operating on the head and neck more." Most had not been exposed to this specialty while in medical school.

Specifically, the appeal was in the wide variety of problems and the opportunity ". . . to work intensively in medical and surgical areas with all age groups."

Otolaryngologists report that they, similar to other surgeons, would not want to practice psychiatry: "scientific base not well founded"; pediatrics: "all office-based"; or pathology: "no people contact."

What Do You Like Most About Otolaryngology?

"Many of the patients we see can be diagnosed on physical findings, i.e., an astute exam of the head and neck is more important than lab data in many instances"; "ability to solve problems finitely"; "I rarely have to care for really sick people"; "technical challenges"; "variety"; "surgical correction of problems"; and "interaction with patients."

A statistically significant percentage of physicians in this specialty report that they are "dissatisfied" (25.2 percent) with only 38.8 percent indicating "very satisfied." [4]

What Do You Like Least About Otolaryngology?

Respondents cite "paperwork" and other aspects of managing an office (as do almost all of the contributors to this book) as the least-liked aspect of their practice. One respondent does not like "night trauma" or "emergencies" and another dislikes "nosebleeds." On a different level one respondent least liked "The fact that some of my colleagues in other specialties are not very knowledgeable about what an otolaryngologist–head and neck surgeon can do. For example, we perform about 90 percent of the head and neck cancer surgery and about 50 percent of the cosmetic and reconstructive surgery of the head and neck."

What Is Your Typical Daily Schedule?

Some otolaryngologists divide their weeks into surgery days and office days. Others spend their mornings operating and their afternoons in the office. Although it is difficult to maintain skills in all aspects of otolaryngology, all the respondents report treating a variety of problems. Generally, they see from 25 to 30 patients a day, half of which are follow-up visits. Most work from 10 to 12 hours per day and have on-call schedules that vary with the type of practice setting. For example, in a four-person group, each physician is on call every fourth night and weekend. In addition, there are time commitments to hospital staff and committee meetings.

What Abilities and Talents Are Important in Otolaryngology?

Manual dexterity and the ability to deal with spatial relationships are important. As in ophthalmology, microscopic surgery is performed and, if one does plastic surgery, a good artistic sense is needed.

This specialty requires expertise in the anatomy of the head and neck region as well as an ability "to think physiologically and to have a 'mind's eye' of the surgical anatomy involved."

It is helpful to develop good communication skills: "people cannot see their problems and we have to draw pictures and explain procedures clearly."

What Personality Traits Best Characterize Otolaryngologists?

In temperament, the otolaryngologist is "action-oriented," "decisive," and "perfectionistic." They prefer to deal with problems that can be solved quickly and afford immediate feedback. Other traits are "independence," "aggressive without being rude," and "an open, questioning mind." The Myers-Briggs Type Indicator data [5] show that the same personality types are attracted to both ophthalmology and otolaryngology, with those choosing ophthalmology more patient-oriented and those choosing otolaryngology more technically oriented.

What Advice Would You Give a Medical Student Interested in Otolaryngology?

Because the competition is so stiff for a residency position, it is important to make good grades and get to know the faculty in your school's department. Attend conferences in the otolarynogology department, do research and publish if possible.

Those interested in otolaryngology "should be interested in attaining a high level of manual dexterity since it will be necessary to devote much time to perfecting techniques in various procedures."

What Are the Future Challenges to Otolaryngology?

All respondents cite the technological challenges: satisfactory treatment of neurosensory hearing loss, dizziness, the continuing evolution of the treatment of head and neck cancer, refinement of the treatment of nasal allergy, and advances in neurotology cancer surgery and reconstruction.

A few allude to "developing relations with associated specialties." Otolaryngology overlaps many specialties and, in this time of medical competition, serious problems can arise. Struggles with plastic surgeons over who will perform facial cosmetic operations [6] have led to hospital privilege battles and even courtroom battles. Depending on the geographic location, the otolaryngologist may be frustrated by overlapping areas of not just plastic surgery, but also allergy, thoracic surgery, and pulmonary medicine.

REFERENCES

1. Coombs RH, Vincent CE. *Psychosocial aspects of medical training.* Springfield, IL: Charles C. Thomas Publisher, 1971, p. 451.
2. Smith J. Personal communication. Department of Otolaryngology. Oregon Health Sciences University, Portland, OR, 1992.
3. Henkel G. Fill the gap: strategies for addressing the otolaryngology workforce shortage, ENT Today, January 2010.
4. Leigh JP, Kravitz RL, Schembri M, Samuels SJ,, Mobley S. Physician career satisfaction across specialties. *Arch Intern Med* 2002; 162:1577-1584.
5. McCaulley MH. Application of the Myers-Briggs Type Indicator to medicine and other health professions, Monograph I. Gainesville, FL: Center for Applications of Psychological Type, Inc., 1978, p. 244.
6. Crane M. Doctor competition: More battles spill over into court. *Med Eco* 60(18):195–213, 1984.

Job Values Selection of Otolaryngologists

You can complete the questionnaires and obtain your scores for all specialties online at http://www.sdn.net, or compare your job values (as recorded in the Appendix) with the job values of otolaryngologists:

Otolaryngologists' Choices:	My Choices:
1. Working with people	1. _____
2. Decision making	2. _____
2. Working with my hands	3. _____
3. Creativity	4. _____
(there is a tie for second place)	

No one chose: Good income, security, prestige, feedback from others

Summary Profile of Otolaryngologists (derived from questionnaire answers)	My Personal Profile as an Otolaryngologist				
They tend to:	I tend to: (circle one number)				
	Never	Rarely	Sometimes	Frequently	Always
Enjoy taking care of people	1	2	3	4	5
Become bored with repetitive activity	1	2	3	4	5
Have manual dexterity	1	2	3	4	5
Need to see tangible results of their efforts quickly	1	2	3	4	5
Prefer a planned schedule	1	2	3	4	5
Act decisively	1	2	3	4	5
Be adventurous/like challenges	1	2	3	4	5
Be objective	1	2	3	4	5
Be "doers" rather than talkers	1	2	3	4	5
Be perfectionistic	1	2	3	4	5

Add total of numbers circled to get your TOTAL SCORE: _____

Transfer score to the Appendix.

Otolaryngology – head and neck surgery

sounds like me _____

could be a possibility _____

doesn't sound like me at all _____

Pathology

FAST FACTS:

Number of first year residency positions offered in the NRMP in 2011 : 518

Filled with US grads in 2011: 51.9 %

Competitiveness: Low - applicants have: an elective in anatomic or clinical pathology, research experience

Length of training: 3-4 years

Number of residency programs: 155

Number of residents in training: 2,212

Competitiveness Rank: Low

Selection criteria for interview/ranking: published medical school research, class rank, grade in senior elective in specialty.

US senior matched applicants' mean Step 1 score: 227

US senior matched applicants' mean Step 2 score: 230

Number in US Board Certified in specialty: 14,127

Median compensation for all physicians in clinical practice: $252,000

Average work hours per week: 45

"THE PATHOLOGIST, I AM CONVINCED, IS THE UNKNOWN man of medicine."[1] Often called "the doctor's doctor," the pathologist acts as consultant to clinicians; therefore the only channels by which his or her services reach the patient are controlled by other doctors.

Some medical students characterize the pathologist as being a "recluse—insecure, uncomfortable, ill at ease with others, and inept in interpersonal communication." Others see the pathologist as "simply trying to beat the hassles of everyday medical practice."[2] All seem to agree, however, that the pathologist prefers the science of medicine over patient care and this specialty offers the physician the opportunity to serve as the link between basic science and clinical medicine.

Pathology is the branch of medicine concerned with the cause, manifestation, diagnosis, and outcome of disease. The pathologist provides the morphologic and laboratory analysis to assist in patient care. Although many pathologists have traditionally practiced both anatomic and clinical pathology, increasingly the trend is to limit one's practice to one or the other area of investigation. An anatomic pathologist's work, often done in a hospital setting, is related to the effects of disease on the human body, for example, the examination of tissues removed from surgical patients and the performance of autopsies. A clinical pathologist specializes in laboratory medicine which includes chemistry, hematology, microbiology, and immunology. The pathologist selects testing methods and equipment, supervises the technical staff, maintains quality control, and confers with clinicians regarding the significance of the tests.

Residency Information. A combined anatomic and clinical pathology residency, preparing physicians for the general practice of pathology requires four years; a single area – anatomic or clinical – requires three years. There is training in medical informatics and management as part of the residency, anticipating that many pathologists may someday direct large laboratories.

Board Certification. Following completion of a residency training program and successful passage of a written examination, one may be certified in anatomic or clinical pathology or both.

Special qualification certificates can be attained in more than 20 subspecialties including the following: blood banking/transfusion medicine, chemical pathology, cytopathology, dermatopathology, forensic pathology, hematolopathology, medical microbiology, molecular diagnostics, neuropathology, and pediatric pathology.

Supply and Projections. A shortage is predicted because growth in this field has been slow.

Economic Status and Types of Practice. An influx of foreign medical graduates in pathology in the 1970s brought increased competition and a drop in income. Many pathologists' expenses are paid for by their hospital employers, third-party payment is received for services rendered, and technicians are employed to help provide services.

The dominant mode of practice has been in a hospital-based setting. However, pathologists also can join a private group practice that may run the hospital laboratory under an exclusive contract and be compensated on the basis of laboratory revenue, per-test fees, or a negotiated salary. Pathologists report that there is increasing competition from large commercial laboratories that do not use the services of pathologists and charge less to perform automated clinical tests.

Other work settings for pathologists include state and local law enforcement agencies, public health departments, medical research centers in the private and public sectors, and academic institutions.

Further Information. The College of American Pathologists, 325 Waukegan Road, Northfield, IL 60093. Telephone: (800) 323-4040. Internet address: www.cap.org.

The American Society of Clinical Pathologists, 2100 West Harrison St., Chicago, IL 60612. Telephone: (312) 738-1336. Internet address: www.ascp.org. Free membership is available for students.

Intersociety Council for Pathology Information, Inc., a non-profit educational organization sponsored by national pathology organizations publishes the Directory of Pathology Training Programs and the brochure Pathology as a Career in Medicine. Accessed at www.pathologytraining.org

A COMPOSITE PICTURE OF THE PATHOLOGIST
Why Choose Pathology?

In choosing this specialty, respondents reported a strong influence by pathologist teachers or research mentors; the initial appeal of pathology involved both the opportunity to do research and the minimal patient contact.

Pathologists' reactions to other specialties include: psychiatry, "too futile"; obstetrics, "too unpredictable"; pediatrics or internal medicine, "patient responsibility and not scientific enough."

What Do You Like Most About Pathology?

Once in practice, pathologists enjoy "the challenge of a difficult case," "the ability to organize tasks," and "conferring with colleagues in different specialties." Also cited as an advantage is the predictable and regular work schedule.

What Do You Like Least About Pathology?

"Administrative problems—being held responsible for situations over which I have no control, such as lab requisitions getting lost, lab work not charted properly"; "nonproductive meetings"; "increasing government regulations"; and "the inability to concentrate on any one task." These responses all indicate that the frustrations in pathology come from not being able to control the environment in which one works to the extent one would like. In addition, pathologists need to obtain more clinical information from physician colleagues to enable better resolution of diagnostic problems.[4]

What Is Your Typical Daily Schedule?

Pathologists tend to have regular schedules, but work hours depend on the type of practice. In a hospital setting the pathologists are tied to the habits of clinicians and because of the heavy involvement with surgeons, may start the day at 7:30 AM and work through to 5:30 PM five days a week, and 7:30 AM to 12:00 PM on Saturdays. They may have night and weekend telephone consultations, but rarely have to return to the hospital. One pathologist says, "In my case, I have duties in practice—looking at surgical pathology and bone marrow materials, seeing to the administration of the laboratories, teaching house staff and medical students, dealing with personnel problems, consulting for federal and private groups, travel on scientific and administrative matters, serving on committees, writing, reading the literature."

Pathologists attend and conduct many meetings because they are called upon to teach and perform consultations for the hospital staff and also to continue the medical education of practicing physicians in the community.

What Abilities and Talents Are Important in Pathology?

A strong scientific orientation with interest in anatomy and histology is basic to pathology. The nature of the work requires the pathologist to have a systematic approach to problems and to have a sense of thoroughness—"a basic trait of an interest in detail and accuracy." Laboratory directors need good management skills.

What Personality Traits Best Characterize Pathologists?

Some pathologists describe themselves as "compulsive," "serious people—somewhat aloof," "studious," and "sort of a blend of the personality traits of engineers and biologists." Another says that pathologists represent a "wide spectrum of human personalities." "People skills" are "invaluable to me as a teacher, interacting with large numbers of laboratory technologists or conferring hourly with clinicians."[3]

What Advice Would You Give a Medical Student Interested in Pathology?

"If you are interested in the scientific aspects of medicine and do not need the ego gratification that comes from patients, pathology should appeal. Because your 'patients' are other physicians for the most part, you still must have a variety of bedside manners, but perhaps a more scientifically sophisticated sort."

While in medical school, students are advised to "develop a fundamental understanding of basic pathologic processes" and to do a research project. In choosing a residency, students are advised to find a program that "caters to the individual's interests. Don't go to a place which features research if your interests are to provide service."

What Are the Future Challenges to Pathology?

Technological and laboratory innovations, such as the ability to explore the molecular origins of disease make this an exciting time to be a pathologist.

However, one respondent says, "Pathology is in a squeeze between governmental and administrative types on one side and physicians who feel threatened on the other." There is a belief that reimbursement practices have adversely affected the specialty and that there is danger of losing their freedom as private practitioners.

The College of American Pathologists has launched a multiyear campaign to "transform the specialty." The goal is to "strengthen and defend the value proposition (i.e., unique benefits) that pathologists offer to patients and fellow clinicians." [4]

REFERENCES

1. German WM. *The story of laboratory medicine.* New York: Duell, Sloan and Pearce, 1941, Preface.

2. Coombs RH. *Mastering medicine.* New York: The Free Press, 1978, pp. 199–200.

3. Lembke A. A piece of my mind. A letter from the Foreign Legion. *JAMA* 1996;276(21):1974.

4. Transforming pathologists. Accessed December 29, 2011. www.cap.org/app/deocs/membership/transformation/new/transform_index.html.

Job Values Selection of Pathologists

You can complete the questionnaires and obtain your scores for all specialties online at http://www.sdn.net, or compare your job values (as recorded in the Appendix) with the job values of pathologist respondents below:

Pathologists' Choices:	My Choices:
1. Decision making	1._____
2. Variety	2._____
3. Independence	3._____
4. Working with my mind	4._____
4. Good income	
4. Creativity	
(there is a three-way tie for fourth place)	

No one chose: Security, prestige, working with my hands

Summary Profile of Pathologists (derived from questionnaire answers)	My Personal Profile as a Pathologist				
They tend to:	I tend to: (circle one number)				
	Never	Rarely	Sometimes	Frequently	Always
Ask why	1	2	3	4	5
Pay attention to details	1	2	3	4	5
Like complex problem solving	1	2	3	4	5
Need control over a situation	1	2	3	4	5
Value independence highly	1	2	3	4	5
Prefer a planned schedule	1	2	3	4	5
Act decisively	1	2	3	4	5
Like to organize people	1	2	3	4	5
Be uncomfortable with poorly defined problems	1	2	3	4	5
Think logically	1	2	3	4	5

Add total of numbers circled to get your TOTAL SCORE: _____

Transfer score to the Appendix.

Pathology

sounds like me _____

could be a possibility _____

doesn't sound like me at all _____

Pediatrics

FAST FACTS:

Number of first year residency positions offered in the NRMP in 2011 : 2,482

Filled with US grads in 2011 : 71.2%

Length of training: 3 years

Number of residency programs: 188

Number of residents in training: 8,124

Competitiveness: Medium

Selection criteria for interview/ranking: grades in required clerkships, grades in senior electives in pediatrics, class rank.

US senior matched applicants' mean Step 1 score: 219

US senior matched applicants' mean Step 2 score: 229

Number in US Board Certified in specialty: 52,270

Starting median compensation: $130,000

Median compensation for all physicians in specialty: $200,000

Average work hours per week: 54

ALMOST ALL MEDICAL STUDENTS HAVE SOME KNOWLEDGE of this specialty because many have been patients of pediatricians. Coombs[1] found that only 12 percent of the first-year medical students in his study did not have a clear impression of pediatrics.

Pediatrics is concerned with the physical, mental, and emotional health of young people from birth to adolescence. It is, therefore, not surprising that the image of the pediatrician is of a person who likes children. One student says, "It's an inner feeling for children that enables them to understand and communicate with little kids who usually make more noise than sense to others."[1] In addition to providing preventive health care, pediatricians are trained to handle acute and chronic illness. However, more and more, children requiring hospitalization are being referred to physicians who have had pediatric subspecialty training.

Residency Information. A residency in general pediatrics is three years in length, encompassing both hospital and ambulatory care experience. After completion of a pediatric residency, an additional two to three years may be taken in the subspecialty area of allergy/immunology. After two years of a pediatric residency, you may begin training in pediatric neurology. An increasing number of residents are choosing to subspecialize in two- to three-year programs.[2] There are also combined internal medicine-pediatrics, pediatrics-emergency medicine, pediatrics-physical medicine and rehabilitation, and pediatric psychiatry–child psychiatry programs.

There has been an increase in applications for the first-year pediatric positions offered each year through the National Resident Matching Program.

Board Certification. Upon successful completion of three years of a pediatrics residency you may apply to take the written examination. There are multiple subspecialty areas of pediatrics: adolescent medicine, cardiology, child abuse pediatrics, critical care medicine, developmental-behavioral pediatrics, emergency medicine, endocrinology, gastroenterology, hematology-oncology, hospice and palliative care, infectious diseases, medical toxicology, neonatal-perinatal medicine, nephrology, neurodevelopmental disabilities, pulmonology, rheumatology, transplant hepatology, sleep medicine, and sports medicine.

There is a special agreement between the American Board of Pediatrics and the American Board of Internal Medicine that enables you to fulfill the training requirements of both Boards by completing two years of training in pediatrics and two years in internal medicine. There are about 100 combined medicine/pediatrics programs. There is also a special agreement between the American Board of Pediatrics and the American Board of Psychiatry and Neurology that enables you to fulfill the training requirements of both Boards by completing two years of training in pediatrics and the neurology training necessary to meet the requirements for certification in neurology with special qualification in child neurology. Another agreement exists between the American Board of Pediatrics and the American Board of Emergency Medicine for certification in both specialties.

Supply and Projections. There is concern that with the aging population and the large number of pediatricians under the age of 45, there will be a serious oversupply of general pediatricians. From 1970 to 1996 there was a 191 percent increase in the number of pediatricians while at the same time, only a 5.4 percent increase in children ages 0–20. Pediatricians in practice have concerns about allied health professionals and family physicians also providing care for children. There is a great need for better geographic distribution of pediatricians to serve rural and inner-city populations. An updated Pediatrician Workforce Statement [2] concludes that "the current pediatric workforce seems adequate to meet the health needs of US children, although significant regional variations may result in local shortages or oversupply, and subspecialty gaps remain to be addressed." In addition, efforts to provide health insurance for all children and a pattern of pediatricians working part-time (24.1 percent in 2009 [3]) may influence the projections.

Economic Status and Types of Practice. General pediatricians are at the low end of the income scale. Increasing time in practice is spent in psychosocial counseling and preventive medicine, which are not well reimbursed services. Pediatric subspecialists, particularly those in the procedural subspecialties, have higher incomes. Current median compensation for pediatric gastroenterology is $165,094 and for pediatric cardiology is $185,000.

Most pediatricians are in private practices located in medium- to large-size cities. They tend to practice in locations with a high per capita income.[3] There are opportunities for pediatricians to work in community, state, or national public health agencies. Many subspecialists pursue academic careers, combining patient care with teaching and research.

Further Information. The American Academy of Pediatrics, 141 Northwest Point Road, P.O. Box 927, Elk Grove Village, IL 60007. Telephone: (847) 434-4000 or (800) 433-9016. Internet address: www. aap.org. Information on a pediatrics career and residency is available at the website.

American College of Osteopathic Pediatricians, 5301 Wisconsin Avenue NW, Suite 630, Washington, DC 20015. Telephone: (202) 686-1700.

A COMPOSITE PICTURE OF THE PEDIATRICIAN
Why Choose Pediatrics?

The appeal of pediatrics is in working with a growing and developing population rather than with people who have problems related to "degeneration, unhealthy lifestyle, or social pathology." One respondent says, "I hate death and the futility of trying to patch people up. I enjoy the building and creativity of kids."

The decision to be a pediatrician is often made early, either before or during medical school. In a survey [4] of more than 500 residency applicants, almost half cited work done with children before medical school as the strongest influence in their specialty choice. Role models are often a factor in this decision: "The chief of pediatrics at a local community hospital was a great teacher and still loved what he did after 30 years of practice." The word "fun" is used to describe the student clerkship in pediatrics.

Pediatricians report that they would not want to practice family medicine because it is "too broad—I could never feel competent"; internal medicine because "I don't want to work with elderly ill patients—it's too depressing"; radiology or pathology because there isn't enough patient contact; surgery because it is "too time demanding," doesn't have enough intellectual challenge, and "the technology separates the physician from the patient"; and emergency medicine because "the contact with patients is too brief and superficial."

What Do You Like Most About Pediatrics?

Building relationships with people is enjoyable to pediatricians: "Feedback from families that they trust me, they come back, they refer their friends—it is gratifying." One respondent has "the feeling that I am doing some good in helping kids and families reach more in the direction of their potential." Specifically, the respondent enjoys the fact that "a lot of anticipatory guidance, preventive medicine, health maintenance is stressed, not just intervening in disease." This is quite different from the surgical specialties where the enjoyment most often comes from seeing immediate results of the work performed.

A statistically significant high percentage (48.1 percent) of pediatricians report being "very satisfied" and only "12.6 percent indicate that they are "dissatisfied." [5]

What Do You Like Least About Pediatrics?

Patient education can be frustrating: "Parents have the ingrained belief that drugs will solve everything and I spend a tremendous amount of time educating people in general common sense." Pediatricians also dislike the "financial constraints when dealing with catastrophic illness in children of young families" and "death of a patient."

What Is Your Typical Daily Schedule?

Most of the general pediatrician's work day is spent in office practice. Much time is spent in preventive care, providing immunizations and check-ups for healthy babies and children. Those pediatricians who are expanding into adolescent medicine find that they must spend much time counseling. Often office hours are extended to include evenings and weekends to accommodate the schedules of their patient population. "On-call" schedules vary with the type of practice and community needs, but they are reported to be "busy," primarily involving telephone calls from worried parents.

What Abilities and Talents Are Important in Pediatrics?

In addition to having a natural affinity for children, pediatricians need to be able to "rapidly instill confidence in parents. Parents are harder to convince than children." To do this, the pediatrician needs to be a good listener, well organized, and able to teach and motivate others. One respondent says that pediatricians need "public relations" skills.

In dealing with adolescents it is particularly important to cultivate "an easiness of communication about yourself and be comfortable with your own sexuality."

What Personality Traits Best Characterize Pediatricians?

Pediatricians described themselves as being patient, good natured, sensitive, and "easy going for medical people." They have the ability to accept delayed gratification, unlike the surgeons who prefer to see their results immediately. They enjoy high levels of interpersonal contact and direct care for people. Their sensitivity is expressed by a tolerance for the faults of others: "Pediatricians aren't usually mean to nurses or other hospital personnel."

What Advice Would You Give a Medical Student Interested in Pediatrics?

In addition to "Be sure you feel comfortable around children" is this advice: "Be aware that you deal with parents in nearly all cases." Another respondent says, "Be sure you understand the difference between how children behave when well versus when they are ill, and how much stress parents feel and will exert on the physician when their child is ill. You must be comfortable with the lack of details and specifics in both the history and physical because children cannot or will not be specific or, often, cooperative."

In relationship to practice, students are advised to learn about all the career options in pediatrics—hospital based, private office based, public health, and school health. If choosing private practice, "be prepared to work hard for your income and be creative in seeking ways to practice cost efficiency." One respondent encourages students to develop a subspecialty interest.

What Are the Future Challenges to Pediatrics?

The scope of the specialty has changed as adolescent health is now included in many pediatric practices. There needs to be more emphasis on behavioral counseling and sex education in general pediatric training and practice.

Access to health care for all children, especially in regard to immunizations, and ethical concerns about genetic manipulation are reported as concerns.[6]

REFERENCES

1. Coombs RH. *Mastering medicine.* New York: The Free Press, 1978, p. 195.
2. Committee on Pediatric Workforce. Pediatric workforce statement. *Pediatrics* 2005; 116(1):263–269.
3. Personal /Practice Characteristics of Pediatrician (U.S. only), 2009. American Academy of pediatrics (AAP) Pediatric Survey of Fellows, accessed www.aap.org/womenpeds/December 29, 2011.
4. Carraccio C, Englander R, Baffa JM. Increases in pediatric residency applications. Letters to the editor. *Acad Med* 1998;73(4):353–354.
5. Leigh JP, Kravitz RL, Schembri M, Samuels SJ, Mobley S. Physician career satisfaction across specialties. *Arch Intern Med* 2002; 162:1577-1584.
6. Shapiro BS, Schwarz DF, Ludwig S. Contempo: Pediatrics. Letter to the editor. *JAMA* 1996;271(2):106.

Job Values Selection of Pediatricians

You can complete the questionnaires and obtain your scores for all specialties online at http://www.sdn.net, or compare your job values (as recorded in the Appendix) with the job values of pediatrician respondents below:

Pediatricians' Choices:	My Choices:
1. Working with people	1. _____
1. Creativity	2. _____
2. Sufficient time off	3. _____
2. Variety	4. _____

(there are ties for first and second place)

No one chose: Decision making, prestige, working with my hands, taking care of people

Summary Profile of Pediatricians (derived from questionnaire answers)   **My Personal Profile as a Pediatrician**

They tend to:	I tend to: (circle one number)				
	Never	Rarely	Sometimes	Frequently	Always
Value time off	1	2	3	4	5
Be easy going	1	2	3	4	5
Be outgoing	1	2	3	4	5
Have good listening skills/ interested in listening	1	2	3	4	5
Enjoy being involved in their patients' lives	1	2	3	4	5
Accept schedule disruptions	1	2	3	4	5
Accept long-term outcomes	1	2	3	4	5
Be tolerant of others	1	2	3	4	5
Enjoy teaching people	1	2	3	4	5
Like harmony	1	2	3	4	5

Add total of numbers circled to get your TOTAL SCORE:_____

Transfer score to the Appendix.

Pediatrics

sounds like me_____

could be a possibility _____

doesn't sound like me at all _____

Physical Medicine
and Rehabilitation

Number of first year residency positions offered in the NRMP in 2011: 86

Filled with US grads in 2011 : 48.8%

Number of second year residency positions offered in the NRMP in 2011: 287

Filled with US grads in 2011 : 48.1%

Competitveness: Low

Length of training: 4 years, including a PGY-1 year of an accredited transitional year or in a preliminary medicine or surgery internship. Other acceptable internships are family medicine , pediatrics or a traditional osteopathic internship.

Number of residency programs: 77

Number of residents in training: 1,211

Competitiveness: Low, but varies by geographic location

Selection criteria for interview/ranking: grades in senior elective in specialty, grades in required clerkships, letters of recommendation

US senior matched applicants' mean Step 1 score: 214

US senior matched applicants' mean Step 2 score: 220

Number in US Board Certified in specialty: 5,803

Starting median compensation: $195,000

Median compensation for all physicians in specialty: $225,000

Average work hours per week: 48

NOT ALL MEDICAL SCHOOLS HAVE DEPARTMENTS OF PHYSICAL medicine and rehabilitation; many medical students do not find out about this specialty until after choosing another field. However, as the media focuses on technological innovations for the physically impaired individual, there is more awareness that physicians are directing the rehabilitative intervention, helping patients attain both maximal physical functional capacity and psychosocial adjustment.

The physician who specializes in physical medicine and rehabilitation—the "physiatrist"—is interested in the diagnosis of the disease processes underlying the disability, but focus is on the functional disability itself—that is, evaluation of the patient's level of functioning, design of a treatment program, and management of the rehabilitation team which carries out the program. There is a basic philosophical tenet in this specialty: "The belief that the physician's responsibility does not end when the acute phase of the illness is over or surgery is completed."[1]

Residency Information. Physical medicine and rehabilitation offers four years of training, including one year of integrated internal medicine (or acceptable equivalent). The training is primarily clinical with a minimum of three months in electrodiagnosis. There are combined five-year double-boarded residency training programs with pediatrics and internal medicine.

Osteopathic programs in Manipulative Medicine offer training for two years after internship or one year after completion of a primary care residency.

Board Certification. Full board certification is achieved when both written (Part I) and oral (Part II) examinations are successfully passed. Part I may be taken after the completion of residency and Part II, after an additional year of clinical experience in physical medicine and rehabilitation.

One year fellowships are available in the following sub-specialties: hospice and palliative care, neuromuscular medicine, spinal cord injury medicine, pain medicine, pediatric rehabilitation medicine, and sports medicine.

Supply and Projections. There is a growing need and a shortage of physicians for this specialty.

Economic Status and Types of Practice. Most practice opportunities are hospital-based and salaries compare favorably to those of other medical specialties. A practice can be adapted to one's own personal preference—private solo or group practice, full-time or part-time hospital or clinic practice, or a combination of these. Physiatrists traditionally have been concentrated in major cities, but even community hospitals in less urban areas are establishing departments of rehabilitation medicine. There is a significant shortage of physiatrists in academics, as well as many opportunities in research.

Further Information. The American Academy of Physical Medicine and Rehabilitation,. Telephone: (312) 464-9700. Internet address: www.aapmr.org. The website gives extensive information for medical students about the specialty.

A COMPOSITE PICTURE OF A PHYSIATRIST
Why Choose Physical Medicine and Rehabilitation?
"Breadth (overlaps many specialties), holistic approach, orientation towards patient rather than disease." The specialty is seen as encompassing broad areas of interest and the physiatrist can concentrate on what is most appealing—for example, orthopaedics, neurology, child development, sports medicine, or preventive medicine. The emphasis of physical medicine and rehabilitation is "more than just treating people who are severely disabled"; it involves in-depth and long-term involvement with the "whole person."

The limited number of physiatrists provides an opportunity to impact on the specialty itself; it also enables "a spirit of camaraderie" to exist as well as opportunities "to interact with or even become one of the leaders in the field."

Physiatrists say that they would not want to practice surgery, which is "too much technical work," "too acute," "procedure intensive," "can injure patients too easily"; a field with short-term patient relationships, such as surgery or emergency medicine; specialties with little patient contact (radiology, pathology, anesthesiology); or internal medicine which is "too much disease orientation, not enough emphasis on the person."

What Do You Like Most About Physical Medicine and Rehabilitation?

Patient involvement is the source of satisfaction to physiatrists: "tremendous gratification that my patients are helped greatly," "dealing with people in a comprehensive manner—physical, medical, psychological, social and vocational concerns," "it is conducive to the development of a careful and well-thought-out treatment plan for each patient treated." In particular, physiatrists enjoy the challenge of long-term chronic care and dealing with problems no other specialty deals with.

There is a low percentage (12.6 percent) of those "dissatisfied," but the percentage (39.1 percent) of those "very satisfied" is lower than the total physician percentage (42.3 percent). [3]

What Do You Like Least About Physical Medicine and Rehabilitation?

The administrative aspects were least liked: "frustration with governmental rules/red tape or absence of funds for equipment/procedures for medically indigent disabled," "external forces which influence practice (e.g., changing insurance coverage for therapy)," "the increasing amount of paperwork, which is even more complex and time consuming in rehabilitation, as sources of patient support are reduced."

Some respondents hoped there would be greater knowledge of and appreciation for their specialty by other physicians but, on the whole, physiatrists seem to be among the happiest of physicians concerning their career choice.

What Is Your Typical Daily Schedule?

A physiatrist in private practice will spend part of a typical 8- to 10-hour day participating in hospital rounds and outpatient care. However, as the leader of the rehabilitation team, physiatrists spend a considerable portion of their time supervising team members, coordinating treatment plans, and monitoring implementation of plans. The physiatrist, as the liaison between the rehabilitation team and other specialty physicians, acts as manager of complex, multidisciplinary disorders and is likely to spend part of each day communicating with team members, patients, and their families.

Physiatrists see patients of all ages (although some may wish to pursue specialized areas, such as pediatric rehabilitation). There is a wide range of problems, most commonly with musculoskeletal, circulatory, and nervous system disorders. Some disabilities require local therapeutic measures; a more complicated situation may require rehabilitation involving other health professionals.

On-call duties vary with the practice setting, but generally there are few after-hours calls. One appealing feature of this field is the flexible lifestyle that allows time off for family and other interests.

What Abilities and Talents Are Important in Physical Medicine and Rehabilitation?

In addition to "a solid grounding in anatomy and physiology," the physiatrist needs "an understanding of the psychological processes involved in illness and injury." As the leader of a health care team, good management and listening skills are necessary. Physiatrists must develop the ability to overview the total picture in cases of multifaceted psychological, functional, and medical problems.

It is important to be able to find creative solutions: "Each patient represents a complex singular management challenge." The treatment plan can then be delegated to appropriate specialists.

What Personality Traits Best Characterize Physiatrists?

"Humanistic" qualities are particularly important in this field: being comfortable seeing humanity not always in "perfect" form, doing work that at times is akin to social work/clergy activities, being flexible and open minded, and giving patient care through psychological understanding.

Caring for chronic problems requires a personality that can be content with "small successes over time as opposed to rapid cures."

What Advice Would You Give a Medical Student Interested in Physical Medicine and Rehabilitation?

"Find out how you feel about disabled people. Make sure you enjoy slow change or no change. Spend time in a rehabilitation center and observe speech, occupational, and physical therapies. Fine tune your skills in examination and diagnosis of musculoskeletal and neurological systems. Choose a well-established residency program."

"This is a field that is still undersupplied and one where you can make a large impact."

"I believe that the future belongs with this field: The population is getting older and more and more patients who have disabilities will be in the population for longer periods of time. There is no field that has greater need. This may be especially important to medical students in future years as other specialties become oversupplied."

What Are the Future Challenges to Physical Medicine and Rehabilitation?

This is an exciting time for the specialty as the aging population and technological advances create a growing need for physiatrists. Performing arts medicine—the prevention and treatment of injury and disability incurred by artists, dancers, and musicians—is an emerging area of this specialty. In addition, automation in industry has increased the need for manual workers, such as keyboard data operators, who suffer work-related disorders.[4]

The opportunities for research are numerous: "electrical stimulation for paralyzed patients; special fertility techniques for paraplegics and quadriplegics; advances in knowledge and appreciation of physiology of fitness and exercise; and new technology in equipment; wheelchairs, environmental control systems, synthesized speech."

In an effort to deliver care to disabled and chronically ill people in a time of increasing pressure to hold down costs, there are major shifts in emphasis from inpatient care to on outpatient and day rehabilitation services.[4]

REFERENCES

1. Rusk HA. Quoted in Lane ME. Physical medicine and rehabilitation, a report from the Joint Committee on Graduate Education, American Academy of Physical Medicine and Rehabilitation, Association of Academic Physiatrists, 1983.
2. Leigh JP, Kravitz RL, Schembri M, Samuels SJ,, Mobley S. Physician career satisfaction across specialties. *Arch Intern Med* 2002; 162:1577-1584.
3. DeLisa JA, Jain SS. Physical medicine and rehabilitation. *JAMA* 1991;265(23):3158.
4. Press JM, Lawler MH, Smith JC. Physical medicine and rehabilitation. *JAMA* 1999; 282(10):925-926.

Job Values Selection of Physiatrists

You can complete the questionnaires and obtain your scores for all specialties online at http://www.sdn.net, or compare your job values (as recorded in the Appendix) with the job values of physiatrist respondents below:

Physiatrists' Choices:	My Choices:
1. Working with people	1. _____
2. Creativity	2. _____
2. Taking care of people	3. _____
3. Variety	4. _____
(there is a tie for second place)	

No one chose: Good income, working with my hands, sufficient time off, feedback from others

Summary Profile of Physiatrists (derived from questionnaire answers)	My Personal Profile as a Physiatrist				
They tend to:	I tend to: (circle one number)				
	Never	Rarely	Sometimes	Frequently	Always
Enjoy taking care of people	1	2	3	4	5
Want to help people	1	2	3	4	5
Like complex problem solving	1	2	3	4	5
Enjoy being an "expert"	1	2	3	4	5
Have good listening skills/ interested in listening	1	2	3	4	5
Be adventurous/like challenges	1	2	3	4	5
Like to organize people	1	2	3	4	5
Enjoy being involved in their patients' lives	1	2	3	4	5
Find satisfaction in small gains	1	2	3	4	5
Look for possibilities	1	2	3	4	5

Add total of numbers circled to get your TOTAL SCORE: _____

Transfer score to the Appendix.

Physiatry

sounds like me _____

could be a possibility _____

doesn't sound like me at all _____

Plastic Surgery

FAST FACTS:

Number of integrated residency positions offered in NRMP in 2010: 69

Number of intergrated programs in 2011: 31

Filled with US grads in 2011 : 92.9%

Number of second year positions offered in NRMP in 2011: 38

Filled with US grads in 2011: 89.5%

Number of second year programs: 20

Length of training: Two pathways: independent plastic surgery programs of 2-3 years or integrated programs of 5 -6 years duration.

Number of residents in training: 491

Competitiveness: Very high

Selection criteria for interview/ranking: AOA membership; publications; letters of recommendation from plastic surgeon, especially a friend or colleague; USMLE scores

US senior matched applicants' mean Step 1 score: 245

Number in US Board Certified in specialty: 3,998

Starting median compensation: $285,000

Median compensation for all physicians in specialty: $450,000

Average work hours per week: 58

Of all the fields in medicine, plastic surgery is considered by many to be the most glamorous. It is a field that reflects today's demand for perfection and preoccupation with youthfulness. However, most plastic surgeons do not concentrate solely on cosmetic surgery. Their work involves the repair and correction of congenital defects, trauma surgery, and cancer reconstruction. In many cases the aim is to restore physical function as well as physical appearance.

Residency Information. The traditional path has been to take three years of training in general surgery, followed by two years of plastic surgery. However, some plastic surgery residencies are three years in length, and there is a trend to complete even a five-year surgical residency prior to the plastic surgery training years. Application for plastic surgery training is through the San Francisco Match that takes place in May to start plastic surgery training in July of the following year. All programs will take applicants who have completed training in orthopedic surgery and otolaryngology programs, as well as general surgery.

As a fourth-year medical student, you may apply through the National Residency Matching Program for an integrative pathway – a combined program of three years general surgery and three years plastic surgery.

Fellowships after residency are offered in hand surgery, craniofacial surgery, microsurgery, burn surgery and plastic surgery within the head and neck.

Board Certification. Completion of at least three years of general surgery, an entire otolaryngology or orthopaedic surgery residency plus at least two years of training in plastic surgery are required for admission to the written examination for certification. Following successful passage of the written test and two years of independent practice, you may take the oral examination. A subspecialty certificate in hand surgery is available.

Supply and Projections. In 2006 more than 16 million plastic surgery procedures were performed in the U.S.[1] This, coupled with increasing public acceptance of "the power to change yourself, " has proved previous predictions of a surplus in this specialty to be overstated. One-fourth of plastic surgeons practice in California or New York. The Plastic Surgery Workforce Task Force report concludes that with a significant number of plastic surgeons approaching retirement and an unchanged number of plastic surgery residency training programs, there will be not be enough appropriately trained physicians to meet demand in the next 10 to 15 years. [2]

Economic Status and Types of Practice. The plastic surgeons who mostly perform cosmetic surgery have the highest income levels. The great majority of plastic surgeons are in solo private practice.

Further Information. The American Society of Plastic and Reconstructive Surgeons, 444 East Algonquin Road, Arlington Heights, IL 60005. Telephone:847-228-9900. Internet address: www. plasticsurgery.org.

A COMPOSITE PICTURE OF THE PLASTIC SURGEON

Why Choose Plastic Surgery?

"Plastic surgery is the discipline of creation" and, as such, appeals to the physician who has an artistic nature. All respondents cited the creativity afforded by plastic surgery: "I am able to plan and develop procedures." Another enjoys the "fine, delicate work." In addition, there is a strong appeal in "changing peoples' lives for the better."

Most physicians chose plastic surgery during their internship or residency years. Many had considered other surgical specialties, but had found them "not challenging enough" (obstetrics) or having "depressing results" (neurosurgery). One respondent would not want to practice psychiatry because "I am too impatient to see the results of my intervention"; another says "I would not want to be in any hospital-based practice such as emergency medicine, radiology, or anesthesiology, for you are at the whim of others." It seems that the appeal of plastic surgery includes tangible results in a creative and independent setting.

What Do You Like Most About Plastic Surgery?

As might be expected from the previous section, plastic surgeons report they primarily enjoy the "challenges of reconstruction" and "visible results." Also mentioned are "good results," "variety," "operative procedures," and "few deaths." One respondent enjoys "seeing a problem, planning a strategy, and then following that strategy using my learned skills to solve that problem."

The "very satisfied" responses are reported to be slightly higher (43.3 percent) than the total physician percentage (42.3 percent), but the "dissatisfied" response percentage (23.1 percent) is also higher than the total physician percentage (17.6 percent). [3]

What Do You Like Least About Plastic Surgery?

In a field with such emphasis on the "visible results," it is not surprising that what is least enjoyable are "demanding, ungrateful patients" and "patients who expect too much." Additionally, they cite "insoluble problems" which may be related to the high expectations of patients. As with other specialties, plastic surgeons also experience the frustration of "paperwork" and "hospital politics."

What Is Your Typical Daily Schedule?

Plastic surgeons report a long working day, averaging from 10 to 12 hours. They spend from five to eight hours each day in surgery, and the rest of the time in office practice. Respondents report a variety of activities: care of burns, treatment of congenital disorders, hand surgery, treatment of head and neck tumors, as well as aesthetic surgery. They generally have a patient population ranging from infants to the elderly, although one respondent has a special interest in breast surgery which limits the age and sex of the patient population. Another who does only cosmetic surgery has a patient population of 70 percent women and 30 percent men. American Society of Plastic Surgeons' data [2] report that the top cosmetic surgical procedures in 2001 were nose reshaping, liposuction, eyelid surgery, breast augmentation and facelifts.

Depending on the type of practice and geographic location, a plastic surgeon may be on call for only his or her own postoperative patients or may also be called by the emergency room, "answering calls at any time of the day or night."

What Abilities and Talents Are Important in Plastic Surgery?

Most often cited are artistic abilities and talents: "an eye to appreciate beauty—to see and judge proportions properly," "a concept of spatial relationships," and "attention to fine detail." Plastic surgeons should have "hand-eye coordination," "imagination," "knowledge of anatomy," and "common sense."

What Personality Traits Best Characterize Plastic Surgeons?

Plastic surgeon respondents most often characterize themselves as "perfectionists." Likewise, they also cite being compulsive and meticulous as common traits. They have "a need for applause and admiration," and are "sensitive," which makes their frustration with demanding, ungrateful patients understandable. One respondent sees plastic surgeons as "adaptable" and another is "willing to try new things."

What Advice Would You Give a Medical Student Interested in Plastic Surgery?

"If you don't genuinely care for people, if your objective is 'the good life' rather than one of devotion to those who are deformed or hurt, if you are more concerned with 'the glamorous image' of the plastic surgeon rather than the tremendous amount of dedication and drudgery necessary to achieve the goal—stay away!" Plastic surgery has one of the longest training periods in medicine and respondents warn that the field is "oversaturated, especially in large cities." However, another respondent says, "I believe there is a large need for plastic surgeons since there is a geographic maldistribution in our specialty. Furthermore, the range of problems is so vast that our specialty allows many subspecialties."

What Are the Future Challenges to Plastic Surgery?

One theme among respondents has unanimous agreement: "an exciting horizon of solutions to reconstruction problems not yet dreamed of, whose only limits are imagination and daring." Areas of future challenge include microsurgery and its applications to transplantation surgery, artificial skin for burn patients, and the physiology of scar formation and biochemistry.

Economic constraints create serious problems for academic plastic surgery, which must compete for patients with other specialists and community-based plastic surgeons, including graduates of the program. In the 1990s Congress supported mandatory insurance coverage for breast reconstruction patients and plastic surgeons are currently working to have treatment of children's deformities covered by insurance plans. [4]

REFERENCES

1. Schnur P, Hait P. The History of Plastic Surgery, ASPS and PSEF, Accessed on December 29, 2011 at www.plasticsurgery.org

2. Rohrich RJ, McH+Grath MH, Lawrence WT, Ahmad J. American Society of Plastic Surgeons Plastic Surgery Workforce Task Force: Assessing the plastic surgery workforce: a template for the future of plastic surgery. Plast Reconstr Surg; 2010 Feb; 125(2):736-746.

3. Leigh JP, Kravitz RL, Schembri M, Samuels SJ, Mobley S. Physician career satisfaction across specialties. *Arch Intern Med* 2002; 162:1577-1584.

4. Miller SH. Competitive forces and academic plastic surgery. *Plast Reconstr Surg* 1998;101(5):1389–1399.

Job Values Selection of Plastic Surgeons

You can complete the questionnaires and obtain your scores for all specialties online at http://www.sdn.net, or compare your job values (as recorded in the Appendix) with the job values of plastic surgeon respondents below:

Plastic Surgeons' Choices:	My Choices:
1. Creativity	1. _____
2. Working with people	2. _____
3. Working with my hands	3. _____
3. Independence	4. _____
(there is a tie for third place)	

No one chose: Security, prestige, sufficient time off, feedback from others.

Summary Profile of Plastic Surgeons (derived from questionnaire answers)	My Personal Profile as a Plastic Surgeon				
They tend to:	I tend to: (circle one number)				
	Never	Rarely	Sometimes	Frequently	Always
Pay attention to details	1	2	3	4	5
Want to help people	1	2	3	4	5
Value independence highly	1	2	3	4	5
Have manual dexterity	1	2	3	4	5
Need to see tangible results of their efforts quickly	1	2	3	4	5
Be adventurous/like challenges	1	2	3	4	5
Be energetic/have a high energy level	1	2	3	4	5
Be perfectionistic	1	2	3	4	5
Look for possibilities	1	2	3	4	5
Seek approval	1	2	3	4	5

Add total of numbers circled to get your TOTAL SCORE: _____

Transfer score to the Appendix.

Plastic surgery

sounds like me _____

could be a possibility _____

doesn't sound like me at all _____

Preventive Medicine

DISEASE PREVENTION AND HEALTH PROMOTION IN MEDICINE receive increased emphasis as economic forces dictate a shift away from curing illness to maintaining health. Preventive medicine had a historic impact on the improvement of health for large groups of people in areas such as sanitation and immunization. Today, individuals are becoming interested in behavior change, bringing preventive medicine into the medical marketplace and physician's office.

The three major specialty areas in preventive health are aerospace medicine, occupational medicine, and public health and general preventive medicine.

Aerospace Medicine

FAST FACTS:

Competitiveness: Very high

Length of training: 4 years (primary care or surgery year followed by 3 years in aerospace medicine)

Number of residency programs: 4 (2 military, 2 civilian)

Number of entry level positions: Approximately 40 each year

Selection criteria for interview/ranking: a firm commitment to aerospace medicine, letters of recommendation

Number in US Board Certified in specialty: 203

Income: Varies with setting

Average weekly patient care hours: Varies with setting

Aerospace medicine is a preventive medicine subspecialty whose practitioners focus on the science and art of aviation, space, and environmental medicine. Many people tend to associate this medical field with the military and space program.

Residency Information. There are four residency programs in aerospace medicine: The combined Army/Naval Aerospace and Operational Medical Institute in Pensacola, Florida; the U.S. Air Force School of Aerospace Medicine at Brooks Air Force Base in Texas; The University of Texas Medical Branch Hospitals (NASA) Program at Galveston, Texas; and a civilian program at Wright State University School of Medicine, Dayton, Ohio. Interested students need to finish a year of clinical training involving direct patient care prior to beginning their specific training in aerospace medicine.

Board Certification. The Traditional Residency Pathway includes three years of training in aerospace medicine are required: a clinical year, a year of special training or research in aerospace medicine (teaching and practice may qualify too) for those without residency training in aerospace medicine, and completion of a master's degree in public health or preventive medicine (usually a year's duration). The applicant must have engaged in the study or practice of aerospace medicine for at least two of the five years preceding application for certification.

In April 2010 the American Board of Preventive Medicine (ABPM) announced a new educational pathway to board certification called the Complementary Pathway. It is designed for the mid-career physician who wishes to make a career change into the practice of preventive medicine and achieve certification in one of its three specialty areas – Aerospace Medicine, Occupational Medicine or Public Health and General Preventive Medicine.

Supply and Projections. Aerospace medicine is included in the category of "Preventive Medicine" in workforce studies—a category that is projected to have a shortage of physicians. The AMA data show a decrease in the numbers of physicians who self-identify themselves in this specialty from 1,188 in 1970 to 473 in 2000. In recent years some physicians have become double-boarded and may be practicing another specialty, such as occupational medicine, as their primary field.

Economic Status and Types of Practice. Approximately half of the aerospace medicine physicians serve in the Army, Navy, or Air Force; one-fourth are employed by the Federal Aviation Administration (FAA) or National Aeronautics and Space Administration (NASA); and the balance are employed by industry, the airlines, or are in private practice. One respondent said "This is definitely not the specialty for making a lot of money."

Further Information. The Aerospace Medical Association, 320 South Henry Street, Alexandria, VA 22314. Telephone: (703) 739-2240. Internet address: www.asma.org.

A COMPOSITE PICTURE OF THE AEROSPACE MEDICINE PHYSICIAN

Why Choose Aerospace Medicine?

Physicians often are first introduced to aerospace medicine after the completion of medical school while serving in the military. However, one respondent had decided on a career in aerospace medicine prior to medical school because of a "lifelong interest in aviation."

Rejected were specialties perceived as "repetitive," requiring care of terminally ill patients, or involving a lack of control of personal life.

What Do You Like Most About Aerospace Medicine?

"Every time we think we are ahead of the problems, technology creates new ones, all of them seemingly carrying new hazards for the people whom we serve." Instead of viewing this as a frustration, aerospace medicine physicians find the variety and challenges of their work enjoyable.

What Do You Like Least About Aerospace Medicine?

This is a well-liked field. It seems logical because aerospace medicine physicians are often doing as a paid professional what they consider to be "fun." However, "bureaucracy," "paperwork," "lack of patient care" and "long hours preventing routine schedule for family" were cited as drawbacks.

What Is Your Typical Daily Schedule?

There are no "typical days" in this field. Aerospace medicine may relate to all specialties (even pathology with accident investigations), but it varies according to the type of practice. Physicians in this field may be administrating, teaching, writing, consulting, traveling, performing physical examinations, flying, conducting research, and/or taking care of acute worksite injuries. One physician sees from 25 to 40 individuals in direct patient care in a "typical" 10- to 12-hour day and offers worldwide military and civilian consultations on diving and aircraft accidents. Many report an 8- to 10-hour working day and on-call duties for medical investigation of accidents. Aerospace medicine physicians must maintain flying proficiency; they must also attend continuing medical education sessions.

What Abilities and Talents Are Important in Aerospace Medicine?

Aerospace medicine physicians must integrate medical information from other disciplines. Most problems are not purely medical: "One needs to have full training in physiology, epidemiology, and pathology of environmentally caused medical problems." One respondent says, "What's needed is an above-average grasp of quantitative concepts, statistics, and logic; a mind which enjoys complex problem solving; and an ability to step back from the trees to see the woods. Each of these is required in epidemiologic studies, and it is the discipline of epidemiology that sets preventive medicine apart from the other specialties."

It is also important to actually pilot aircraft so as to understand the stress of flight.

What Personality Traits Best Characterize Aerospace Medicine Physicians?

Although some respondents state that there is no one personality type in aerospace medicine, the Myers-Briggs Type Indicator data suggest that "practical and matter-of-fact" types are attracted to this specialty. The "tough-minded" types most frequently found in engineering are in aerospace medicine.

"Persons who require one-to-one patient contact for ego gratification are apt to be unhappy. The people who have been outstandingly successful in aerospace medicine have been inquisitive, strongly interested in the health sciences, especially physiology, physics, and psychology. Patience is required: One can spend several years working on a single problem."

What Advice Would You Give a Medical Student Interested in Aerospace Medicine?

Recommendations include learning to fly, joining a military scholarship program to get training and basic experience, and examining one's personal need to treat patients because aerospace medicine is basically a preventive rather than treatment-oriented specialty. "If engineering, science, research, and management can be more important than seeing a great number of patients, consider aerospace medicine." Also, "recognize that the thrust of the specialty is toward preventing illness and injury in flyers and passengers."

Students are warned that there are "limited opportunities for full-time employment" and they are advised to "explore all facets of the current practice of aviation medicine before committing to a residency training program." Many respondents said that one should be a fully trained clinician—"seek the best, most diversified teaching internship or first year residency. Thereafter, seek out an excellent master's of public health program for a year; it will do no harm even if one returns to clinical medicine, and it will afford excellent exposure to preventive medicine." One respondent recommended a full residency in a clinical specialty prior to a residency in aerospace medicine.

What Are the Future Challenges to Aerospace Medicine?

"Endless and boundless as long as man flies higher, further, faster, and longer."

Space flight is most often cited as a future challenge. Of special interest is the application of telemedicine, which is used in the space program, to patient care via satellite communications.[1]

In addition, there are the problems associated with aircraft and personnel safety, including air traffic controllers' health, psychological stress on pilots, and treatment for the flying population—flight personnel and passengers.

REFERENCE

1. Rayman RB. Aerospace medicine. Contempo 1998. *JAMA* 1998;279(22):1777–1778.

Job Values Selection of Aerospace Medicine Physicians

You can complete the questionnaires and obtain your scores for all specialties online at http://www.sdn.net, or compare your job values (as recorded in the Appendix) with the job values of aerospace medicine physician respondents below:

Aerospace Medicine Physicians' Choices:	My Choices:
1. Achievement	1. _____
2. Creativity	2. _____
2. Variety	3. _____
2. Working with people	4. _____
(there is a three-way tie for second place)	

No one chose: Good income, working with my hands, taking care of people, feedback from others

Summary Profile of Aerospace Medicine Physicians (derived from questionnaire answers)	My Personal Profile as an Aerospace Medicine Physician

They tend to:

I tend to: (circle one number)

	Never	Rarely	Sometimes	Frequently	Always
Become bored with repetitive activity	1	2	3	4	5
Like complex problem solving	1	2	3	4	5
Be outgoing	1	2	3	4	5
Be adventurous/like challenges	1	2	3	4	5
Tolerate the unknown	1	2	3	4	5
Accept long-term outcomes	1	2	3	4	5
Be energetic/have a high energy level	1	2	3	4	5
Be achievers	1	2	3	4	5
Think logically	1	2	3	4	5
Look for possibilities	1	2	3	4	5

Add total of numbers circled to get your TOTAL SCORE: _____

Transfer score to the Appendix.

Aerospace medicine

sounds like me _____

could be a possibility _____

doesn't sound like me at all _____

Occupational Medicine

FAST FACTS:

Length of training: 3 years (after one clinical residency year)
Number of residency programs: approximately 40
Number of residents in training: 160
Competitiveness: Low
Number in US Board Certified in specialty: 1,003
Starting median compensation: $139,000
Median compensation for all physicians in specialty: $166,273
Average weekly patient care hours: Varies with the setting

Medical students have little formal training in or exposure to occupational medicine, a preventive medicine subspecialty. The focus of this specialty is health in the workplace. Occupational medicine physicians are both clinicians dealing with work-related disease and injury and specialists in environmental hazards advising on ways to protect workers and managers on the job. They have expertise in mechanical stresses, the psychological effects of working conditions, and radiation and toxicology.[1] Originally called "industrial" medicine, the scope was broadened in the 1950s to include all business establishments and today, as occupational medicine physicians concern themselves with other community health problems, some companies are using the term "environmental health."

Residency Information. The length of the programs varies from two to three years. The recommended sequence is a year in a clinical residency program, an academic year which leads to the master of public health degree, and a practicum year of residency with supervised training and field experience in occupational medicine. In some programs, the academic and practicum year are taken together over a two-year period, with time devoted to each.

Board Certification. The American Board of Preventive Medicine offers board certification in occupational medicine. Traditionally, after successful completion of the three years of training or one year in full-time practice, teaching, research, or special training in occupational medicine, you may apply to take the written examination for certification. In addition, you must have been engaged in the training for, or the practice of, occupational medicine for at least two of the five years preceding application for certification.

In April 2010 the ABPM announced a new educational pathway to board certification called the Complementary Pathway. It is designed for the mid-career physician who wishes to make a career change into the practice of preventive medicine and achieve certification in one of its three specialty areas – Aerospace Medicine, Occupational Medicine or Public Health and General Preventive Medicine.

Supply and Projections. Occupational medicine is included in the category of "Preventive Medicine" in workforce studies—a category that is projected to have a shortage of physicians. Physician recruiters are getting requests for family physicians who want to practice occupational medicine because of their focus on preventive as well as curative medicine,[2] a strategy that companies hope will improve productivity.

There are 6,000 members of the American College of Occupational and Environmental Medicine with about 65 percent in clinical practice, 18 percent in administrative roles, and 12 percent serving as consultants. [3] However, many more physicians are employed by companies on a part-time basis.

Economic Status and Types of Practice. Those who are salaried do not have the expense of staffing and operating a private office. Occupational medicine is said to be "one of the last bastions of fee-for-service practice" because you may establish your own occupational medicine clinic.[2]

Opportunities to practice occupational medicine exist in a variety of settings: on a part-time basis with one or more small companies, or full-time in a medium or large organization. Most companies with more than 1000 employees offer some degree of medical service and in a larger organization there is a corporate medical director overseeing a number of staff physicians, nursing personnel, and ancillary or paramedical personnel. In addition, you may be employed by a hospital or university-based occupational medical center, many of which receive funding from the National Institute for Occupational Safety and Health; by a state or federal agency; or by an academic or research institution.

Further Information. The American College of Occupational and Environmental Medicine, 25 Northwest Point Boulevard, Suite 700 Elk Grove Village, IL 60005. Telephone: (847) 818-1800. Internet address: www.acoem.org.

A COMPOSITE PICTURE OF THE OCCUPATIONAL MEDICINE PHYSICIAN

All respondents are employed full time in occupational medicine and are certified by the American Board of Preventive Medicine in the area of occupational medicine.

Why Choose Occupational Medicine?

Most respondents had embarked on careers in other specialties before changing to occupational medicine. One had completed surgical training and, during military service, was assigned to initiate a program in industrial medicine; another found the hours in general practice to be chaotic. Survey results from 151 occupational and environmental residents show that 62 percent entered residencies after practicing other specialties.[4]

The preventive aspects of this specialty are appealing: "The unknown facts about cause and effect and the obvious possibility of developing preventive methods for controlling occupational illnesses and injuries intrigued me and challenged me." Also intriguing is the "opportunity to affect a larger population." One respondent was interested in clinical toxicology and clinical pharmacology, but was interested in the clinical rather than research applications of these fields; another was interested in chest diseases and has become an authority on asbestos-related illnesses. The resident survey[4] affirms the appeal of prevention (64 percent), lifestyle (56 percent), and issues related to workers (53 percent).

What Do You Like Most About Occupational Medicine?

Occupational physicians report they enjoy management challenges: "the challenge of planning, leading, and organizing a large corporate medical program with many physicians, nurses, epidemiologists, and toxicologists working for me."

Patient contact is also important in this specialty: "I have the chance to spend more time with patients—the clock doesn't run." "I enjoy the social aspects, i.e., caring for workers involved in a hazardous occupation."

As in other preventive health care specialties, patient education is involved and respondents report that they enjoy "teaching, a presentation of examples, and continued communication, both orally and in writing, which will allow managers to know what is truly meant by occupational health." "I enjoy the intense effort required to enable managers and workers to appreciate the value of preventive measures."

More physicians in this specialty are "very satisfied" (43.8 percent) and less "dissatisfied" (15.1 percent) than the total percentage of physicians. [5] A more recent survey[6] of a random sample of members of the American College of occupational and Environmental Medicine revealed that 80 percent of the 610 respondents were satisfied with their choice of career. This may reflect the number who enter this field as a career change or to expand their practice. It offers an opportunity for education while learning, as they can take postgraduate short courses, some of which are available through distance learning. [3]

What Do You Like Least About Occupational Medicine?

Frustrations with working within a bureaucracy arise when "management changes frequently," "it is difficult to get programs initiated," "managers are not sensitive to the needs of employees," and "employees try to take advantage of the company by using health as an excuse for attendance or performance problems."

One respondent's work setting affords "fewer opportunities to apply clinical skills" and "a decrease in contacts with other medical colleagues."

What Is Your Typical Daily Schedule?

Occupational medicine offers a variety of daily activities, depending on the type of practice. Some occupational medicine physicians are administrators and do not see patients; some take care of ill and injured employees and offer preventive services; some are engaged in research and/or teaching. The administrator's duties are described: "I am at present responsible for all aspects of medical know-how required by managers, physicians, nurses, and technicians employed by the five manufacturing divisions of the corporation. My duties require reports to be written or reviewed and acted upon; studies of health hazards and epidemiological studies to be designed and periodically reviewed; the interpretation of radiographs; the preparation of product and raw materials safety data sheets for employees, customers' employees, and consumers; and numerous telephone conversations with managers, colleagues, and legal advisers. In order for me to do my job I need to know all about manufacturing processes and the sites where they take place. This necessitates a good deal of travel." Others in administration report time spent reviewing disability and workers' compensation cases, meetings with company management regarding policy guidelines and monitoring of medical service programs, and reading medical journals and literature generated by the company.

Work hours are generally fewer than in other specialties with respondents reporting 8 to 10 hours daily. The work day of those primarily involved in patient care is related to the company work schedule. Some companies have on-call schedules, although this generally involves "telephone consultation with on duty personnel, rather than having to return to the plant." Some occupational medicine physicians have teaching affiliations with medical schools or serve as consultants to local hospitals.

What Abilities and Talents Are Important in Occupational Medicine?

Administrative expertise, writing and speaking skills, and the ability to communicate in a manner understood by employees and management alike are all important in occupational medicine. In addition, you should have interest and good background in the related disciplines of occupational safety, industrial hygiene, epidemiology, and biostatistics.

What Personality Traits Best Characterize the Occupational Medicine Physician?

"Problem solvers" and "people oriented" are traits the respondents use to describe themselves. Problem solving refers both to clinical and management situations: "An insatiable curiosity and inquiring mind are essential." With regard to people, "There must be a sense of justice, with the willingness to speak out when visible harm is being done to an employee, either physically, psychologically, or chemically" and most have "the ability to work as a team member rather than having to be the highly individualized, solo practitioner in an office."

What Advice Would You Give a Medical Student Interested in Occupational Medicine?

Almost all respondents advise specializing first in a clinical field—"Be a good clinician first"—and engaging in private practice for some time prior to formal training in occupational medicine. In addition, one respondent says, "Were I to do it again, I would want much greater grounding in behavioral psychology, psychiatry, and sociology."

Many occupational medicine physicians have had some previous experience with the business world. "Even a summer job in a factory will sensitize you to the problems and opportunities in this specialty."

What Are the Future Challenges to Occupational Medicine?

Respondents view occupational medicine as "a dynamic movement in health care": "Occupational health and safety have made great strides in recent years and are offering opportunities to physicians to participate in the progress." Demand for physicians trained in this specialty far exceeds the supply and the need is expected to continue to grow.

Some optimism comes from industry's desire to control the rising costs of health care delivery and respondents cite challenges to "intervene in lifestyle-caused disease in the work setting." Another challenge is "the shifting emphasis from investigation and treatment of occupational illnesses and injuries to the prevention of the adverse effects from exposure to chemicals and materials in the work environment." Occupational medicine physicians also will be challenged to develop programs that will anticipate and comply with government regulation of the workplace.

REFERENCES

1. American College of Preventive Medicine/Association of Teachers of Preventive Medicine. *Careers in preventive medicine.* Washington, DC, 1984, p. 5.
2. Guardiano JR. Occupational medicine a "team"play. *Fam Pract News* 1998;28(7):57.
3. Brunk D. Occupational medicine can mean job satisfaction. *Fam Pract News* 2002;32(9):44.
4. Schwartz BS et al. Recruiting the occupational and environmental medicine physicians of the future: Results of a survey of current residents. *J Occup Environ Med* 1995;37:739–743.
5. Leigh JP, Kravitz RL, Schembri M, Samuels SJ, Mobley S. Physician career satisfaction across specialties. *Arch Intern Med* 2002; 162:1577-1584.
6. Baker BA, Dodd K, Greaves IA, et al. Occupational medicine physicians in the United states:demographics and core competencies. *J Occup Environ Med;* 2007 Apr;49(4):388-400.

Job Values Selection of Occupational Medicine Physicians

You can complete the questionnaires and obtain your scores for all specialties online at http://www.sdn.net, or compare your job values (as recorded in the Appendix) with the job values of occupational medicine physician respondents below:

Occupational Medicine Physicians' Choices:	My Choices:
1. Decision making	1. _____
2. Creativity	2. _____
2. Variety	3. _____
2. Working with people	4. _____
(there is a three-way tie for second place)	

No one chose: Sufficient time off, prestige, security

Summary Profile of Occupational Medicine Physicians (derived from questionnaire answers)	My Personal Profile as an Occupational Medicine Physician				
They tend to:	I tend to: (circle one number)				
	Never	Rarely	Sometimes	Frequently	Always
Want to help people	1	2	3	4	5
Like complex problem solving	1	2	3	4	5
Be team players	1	2	3	4	5
Prefer a planned schedule	1	2	3	4	5
Act decisively	1	2	3	4	5
Be adventurous/like challenges	1	2	3	4	5
Like to organize people	1	2	3	4	5
Be able to coordinate tasks	1	2	3	4	5
Accept long-term outcomes	1	2	3	4	5
Be warm and sympathetic	1	2	3	4	5

Add total of numbers circled to get your TOTAL SCORE: _____

Transfer score to the Appendix.

Occupational medicine

    sounds like me _____

    could be a possibility _____

    doesn't sound like me at all _____

Public Health and General Preventive Medicine

██████████ **FAST FACTS:** ██████████

Number of first year residency positions offered in the NRMP in 2011: 5 (most positions not in the NRMP)

Length of training: 2 years, if preceded by completion of a clinical residency; 3 years, if directly from medical school. Can be completed in combination with a clinical residency through a 4-5 year dual program.

Number of residents in training: 262

Competitiveness Rank: Low

Selection criteria for interview/ranking: experience in the field by doing an elective, commitment to population based health

Number in US Board Certified in specialty: 442

Average income: Lower than national average of $194,400 for MDs

Average weekly professional hours: Varies with practice setting

Public health and preventive medicine are considered here as one specialty. There is a combined examination for board certification, even though residency training programs may focus on either general preventive medicine or preventive medicine-public health.

The aim of both public health and preventive medicine is ". . . to promote health and understand the risks of disease, injury, disability, and death, seeking to modify and eliminate these risks." [1] While this goal is incorporated into other medical specialties, such as family practice and pediatrics, it is the primary focus of those who choose a preventive medicine specialty. In addition, the preventive medicine physician—whether in aerospace medicine, occupational medicine, or public health and general preventive medicine—will be interested in community efforts for large population groups as well as the health of individual patients.

Residency Information. The three-year residency in preventive medicine or preventive medicine-public health includes a clinical, academic, and practicum year. There are very few first-year positions in preventive medicine residency programs so probably you will need to find a position in a transitional year or in a clinical residency such as family medicine, internal medicine, obstetrics and gynecology, or pediatrics. You then apply directly to programs in preventive medicine specialties during your internship year. During the academic year you will earn a master's degree in either public health or a related discipline, and receive training in biostatistics, epidemiology, environmental health, health services administration, social and behavioral medicine, and in community measures to prevent the occurrence, progression, and disabling effects of disease and injury. For the third year, you will have supervised practical experience in the field.

There are residency programs in public health or general preventive medicine and a few in combined preventive medicine-public health. They may be one to three years in length and are in various settings— schools of public health, medical schools, or county and state health departments. In addition, there are a few four-year programs combined with family medicine or internal medicine.

Subspecialty training is available in medical toxicology and undersea and hyperbaric medicine.

Board Certification. After successful completion of the residency training described above or at least one year in full-time practice, teaching, research, or special training in preventive medicine you may apply to take the written certification examination. In addition, you must have been engaged in the training for, or practice of, preventive medicine for at least two of the five years preceding application for certification.

In April 2010 the ABPM announced a new educational pathway to board certification called the Complementary Pathway. It is designed for the mid-career physician who wishes to make a career change into the practice of preventive medicine and achieve certification in one of its three specialty areas – Aerospace Medicine, Occupational Medicine or Public Health and General Preventive Medicine.

Supply and Projections. Presently about 1800 physicians are self-identified in AMA data as practicing "public health." The AMA does not have a category of "preventive medicine." Public health is described as "a growing, almost limitless field," especially for physicians who earn a master's degree in public health (MPH) or become board-certified in preventive medicine.[2] It is "undersupplied" in all workforce studies.

Economic Status and Types of Practice. Preventive medicine is not a high paying medical specialty, but the income range will vary according to the type of practice chosen. The majority of positions will be salaried, but practice expenses are low or nonexistent because office space, personnel, and liability insurance all are provided by the employer.

Starting positions often require primary care clinical work in local government facilities and agencies. Additional work settings for preventive medicine physicians include local or state health departments, federal agencies such as the Centers for Disease Control and the National Institutes of Health, international agencies such as the World Health Organization, and university medical schools and schools of public health (for research, teaching, and consulting). One respondent is working in undersea medicine in the Navy.

Further Information. The American College of Preventive Medicine, 455 Massachusetts Ave. NW, Suite 200, Washington, DC 200051 Telephone: (202) 466-2044. Internet address: www.acpm.org. The website has information on careers in the specialty.

Undersea and Hyperbaric Medical Society, 10531 Metropolitan Avenue, Kensington, Maryland 20895. Telephone: (301)942-2980. Internet address: www.uhms.org.

A COMPOSITE PICTURE OF THE PUBLIC HEALTH-PREVENTIVE MEDICINE PHYSICIAN

Why Choose Public Health-Preventative Medicine?

Although first introduced to preventive medicine during medical school, many physicians chose other specialties prior to embarking on preventive medicine careers. One respondent left his private practice of internal medicine after seven years because of "the futility of treating patients on a one-to-one basis when the problems are spread so diffusely through society." Another respondent, while serving in the Peace Corps in Nigeria, decided that, "curative medicine was obviously a waste of time, resources, and people."

A few, however, decided on preventive medicine during medical school, finding the "possibility of combining interests in social and political spheres with medical practice." Also alluring was "the status of being a specialist in a field with very few others," "the diversity of opportunities and intellectual stimulation," and "good hours."

Preventive medicine respondents report that they would not want to practice specialties requiring involvement with "intense personal problems of people," such as psychiatry; dealing with dying patients, such as oncology; or focusing on curing rather than preventing illness, such as surgery. Most indicate that they would not want to be in private fee-for-service practice, believing it would be "very narrow and dull compared with the challenges and variety of public health."

What Do You Like Most About Public Health-Preventative Medicine?

Variety and intellectual challenge afford the most enjoyment: "Each day opens new avenues—from establishing a new family planning clinic, building a new health department, taking over the indigent care clinics when the county has cancelled its hospital contract because of the expense, to securing an in-house computer system." There are also "the belief I have that my work contributes to the public's well-being" and "the ability to adjust my schedule to meet my family's needs."

What Do You Like Least About Public Health-Preventative Medicine?

Routine paperwork and dealing with bureaucracy are cited most often. Also mentioned is the trend toward replacing health professionals by administrators, the low level of public and general financial support for work performed, and the lack of status in the medical community. One respondent observes, "Being in the public eye as a 'bureaucrat' makes one subject to all types of criticism, mostly unwarranted. This is not a problem if one sticks to a pure program area, like disease control, but if one runs a public health agency, one is subject to much abuse from the press and the special interest groups."

What Is Your Typical Daily Schedule?

No day is typical in this specialty, but meetings seem to occupy many hours: "We have continual meetings on everything from rats and rabies to air pollution and motorcycle helmet laws. In a public health position, meetings with elected officials at local, state, or national levels are common. Public health, when practiced creatively, has no routine."

Activities can be grouped into categories of teaching, research, administration, meetings, and clinical care with time allocated to those that are appropriate to the practice setting. Generally, preventive medicine specialists work an 8- to 10-hour day and have no formal on-call schedule. However, many report evening meetings with lay and professional groups and time spent after hours on research and writing projects. In addition, "public health administrators are always on call if health crises (floods, etc.) occur." Although most activity occurs in offices or conferences, a considerable amount of national and international traveling is reported.

What Abilities and Talents Are Important in Public Health-Preventative Medicine?

The abilities to synthesize and organize information, do long-term planning, think quantitatively and logically, and convince others to follow your ideas and join you in your work are all important. The art of negotiation and compromise is often necessary, as are speaking and writing skills.

A public health-preventive medicine physician needs a broad medical perspective and "knowledge of public health, environmental, epidemiologic, medicolegal, health financing, health management and health delivery principles and issues." It also helps to develop "an awareness of the ebb and flow of politics." In summary, "an ability to do many things well and coordinate all."

What Personality Traits Best Characterize Public Health-Preventative Medicine Physicians?

Preventive medicine physicians see themselves as self-starters, intellectually curious, and problem solvers. Unlike most other fields, they usually do not have an individual patient with a problem to provide stimulus for action.

They cite "an optimistic view of the possibility of improving human health," "a sense of purpose and probably a somewhat missionary spirit," and "high expectations concerning the effectiveness of their work and a low expectation concerning personal rewards" as characteristics of physicians in this field. They also see themselves as "medical detectives who are comfortable with the unknown." They have the trait of being patient, "realizing that the results desired do not happen overnight or in, at times, several years." Patience is also in evidence as they work with "frustrating political processes." Closely related to being patient is the tenacity of staying with a project, sometimes for many years. They tend to be open-minded, diplomatic, and outgoing in interpersonal relationships.

The Myers-Briggs Type Indicator data report that physicians primarily involved in preventive medicine activities (epidemiologists, researchers) are more tough-minded than the physicians working in public health settings who are more humanistically oriented. Both groups, however, are innovative individuals interested in being change agents in improving health care, rather than managers of existing health care systems.

What Advice Would You Give a Medical Student Interested in Public Health-Preventative Medicine?

Students are advised to get a solid background in clinical medicine before entering preventive medicine specialty training. "Be a good physician first so that you know what you want to prevent." Also, "preventive medicine is such a broad specialty that it is difficult to master until you are mature as a physician."

You can begin as early as college years preparing for this field by working on a campus newspaper, joining a debate team, and having interest in economics and politics. In addition, work in a community health agency with "nonsympathetic, nonphysician managers, administrators, policy makers, and legislators" may help clarify your interest. If possible, gain some international experience. In medical school get a good foundation in epidemiology, statistics, and health financing and become involved with organized medical professional organizations.

Once you have chosen this specialty, "select a specific focus to which you wish to commit yourself." "Be willing to move around a bit from job to job and city to city if you wish to advance." A final word of advice: "Only enter if you have the courage to dream of things that have not been."

What Are the Future Challenges to Public Health-Preventative Medicine?

Managed care has brought attention to the health status of populations, and organizations are making ongoing efforts to bring the public health and medical communities together.[3] Such collaboration, however, poses a challenge according to one respondent: "We must keep prevention and public health alive as specialties and not allow them to be fractionated and subsumed in fragments by clinical specialties." The general consensus is that the "future of American medicine will be in the application of prevention to society and its people—these principles can be applied on one patient after another, or on a community wide basis."

A continuing major challenge is the current system of financing graduate medical education. Because most preventive medicine training takes place in non-hospital settings, most residencies do not receive funds from Medicare or other traditional sources of residency financing.

The most recent challenge to the public health community has come with the threat of bioterrorism and the need to be informed on this topic and educators for the public.

REFERENCES

1. American College of Preventive Medicine. *Careers in preventive medicine.* 1991, p. 1.
2. Hinz CA. The doctor of the people. *Unique Opportunities* 1997;7(4):26–36.
3. Ambrose P. Uniting public health and medicine. Resident forum. *JAMA* 1997; 278(21):1722c.

Job Values of Public Health-Preventive Medicine Physicians

You can complete the questionnaires and obtain your scores for all specialties online at http://www.sdn.net, or compare your job values (as recorded in the Appendix) with the job values of public health-preventive medicine physician respondents below:

Public Health-Preventive Medicine Physicians' Choices:	My Choices:
1. Variety	1. _____
2. Creativity	2. _____
3. Decision making	3. _____
4. Working with people	4. _____
4. Working with my mind	
(there is a tie for fourth place)	

No one chose: Working with my hands, taking care of people, feedback from others

Summary Profile of Public Health-Preventive Medicine Physicians (derived from questionnaire answers)	My Personal Profile as a Public Health-Preventive Medicine Physician

They tend to:	I tend to: (circle one number)				
	Never	Rarely	Sometimes	Frequently	Always
Ask why	1	2	3	4	5
Become bored with repetitive activity	1	2	3	4	5
Like complex problem solving	1	2	3	4	5
Be team players	1	2	3	4	5
Act decisively	1	2	3	4	5
Be adventurous/like challenges	1	2	3	4	5
Be able to coordinate tasks	1	2	3	4	5
Tolerate the unknown	1	2	3	4	5
Accept long-term outcomes	1	2	3	4	5
Be self-starters	1	2	3	4	5

Add total of numbers circled to get your TOTAL SCORE: _____

Transfer score to the Appendix.

Public health-preventive medicine

   sounds like me _____

   could be a possibility _____

   doesn't sound like me at all _____

Psychiatry

████████████ **FAST FACTS:** ████████████

Number of first year residency positions offered in the NRMP in 2011: 1097

Filled with US grads in 2011: 58.3%

Length of training: 4 years

Number of residency programs: 185

Number of residents in training: 4,745

Competitiveness: Low

Selection criteria for interview/ranking: grades in required clerkships, grades in electives in specialty, published medical school research

US senior matched applicants' mean Step 1 score: 216

US senior matched applicants' mean Step 2 score: 221

Number in US Board Certified in specialty: 24,893

Starting median compensation: $185,000

Median compensation for all physicians in specialty: $200,000

Average work hours per week: 48

BECAUSE PSYCHIATRISTS ARE CONCERNED WITH MENTAL AND emotional disorders rather than physical diseases, they are often viewed differently from more biologically oriented physicians. The focus of modern American psychiatry, however, is shifting toward the biologic and behavioral approaches to patients' disorders and away from the psychodynamic or social models.[1] In addition, there are advances in pharmacologic treatments of mental disorders and a renewed unity with neuroscience, giving psychiatry more scientific status.

Many psychiatrists are generalists, but there are different models of treatment—for example, individual or group therapy, a behavioral or psychoanalytic focus.

Residency Information. Programs will have different philosophies, such as biologic, psychoanalytic, psychodynamic, etc., so you need to know what type of training you want. Combined programs with internal medicine, family medicine, pediatrics, and neurology are available. A fellowship in child and adolescent psychiatry can begin any time after the clinical first year but must include at least two years of general psychiatry for both allopathic and osteopathic physicians.

Board Certification. After completion of a psychiatry residency you may apply for the written examination, which tests the applicant in both psychiatry and neurology. The subsequent oral examination deals with clinical skills related to clinical psychiatry only.

You may apply for certification in child and adolescent psychiatry after certification in general psychiatry plus completion of two years of training in child psychiatry. The examination has both written and oral components. There are certificates of added qualifications in geriatric psychiatry, clinical neurophysiology, hospice and palliative care, addiction psychiatry, pain management, and forensic psychiatry.

Supply and Projections. Psychiatry was the fastest growing medical specialty in the late 1940s but the number of U.S. medical students filling psychiatry positions on Match Day has declined from 76% in 1988 [2] to 61.4% in 2010. There has been a strong reliance on international medical graduates to fill vacant positions. A reduction in this group would intensify the predicted shortage of psychiatrists.[3] However, there is an uncertain future for psychiatric hospitals and an increasing number of non-physician professionals offering counseling services.

Economic Status and Types of Practice. Reductions in third-party reimbursement and competition from lay practitioners such as psychologists, pastoral counselors, and social workers have kept income levels for general psychiatrists low. Child psychiatrists have a higher median compensation of $172,107.

There are a variety of practice opportunities in psychiatry: You can practice in an office-based setting, be a salaried staff member of a psychiatric hospital, or engage in research and/or academics. The private practice of psychiatry is declining significantly, with most psychiatrists in group or multispecialty practices. At the same time, the proportion of salaried hospital-, clinic-, and health maintenance organization-based psychiatrists is rising.[4] This change may reflect the increased focus in residency training on biology and short-term techniques coupled with pharmacotherapy rather than "the traditional 50-minute hour as the standard of practice," as well as the uncertainty of private practice for recent graduates with high debt.

If you have a special interest, such as forensic psychiatry, you may become a consultant in criminal proceedings or deal with the treatment and rehabilitation of prisoners. Testifying in court will yield a much higher income than the office-based psychiatrist has.

Further Information. The American Psychiatric Association, 1000 Wilson Boulevard, Suite 1825, Arlington, VA 22209. Telephone: (703) 907-7300. Internet address: www.psych.org.

The American Academy of Child and Adolescent Psychiatry, 3615 Wisconsin Avenue NW, Washington DC 20016. Telephone: (202) 966-7300. Internet address: www.aacap.org. The website has information for students about the specialty.

A COMPOSITE PICTURE OF THE PSYCHIATRIST

All the respondents are board certified in general psychiatry. Comments concerning child psychiatry will be from other referenced sources.

Why Choose Psychiatry?

A nationwide study of first-year psychiatry residents[5] revealed that 57 percent considered a mental health career some time before entering medical school, but only 27 percent thought they would be psychiatrists. Nearly 30 percent planned to be family physicians at the time they entered medical school. The psychiatric clerkship was a strong positive influence in their choice of psychiatry as a specialty. The respondents confirmed this study with all but one selecting psychiatry before or during medical school. They say, "I liked psychiatry lectures best and the faculty interest in students," and "I always enjoyed the humanities. In college I chose a mixture of the sciences along with psychology, sociology, and philosophy. Psychiatry offered a chance to continue the combination." One respondent was talked out of psychiatry by other students, took a year of surgery, and found that "people needed something else besides a knife to alter their lives." Many respondents report that the appeal of psychiatry involved its challenging nature and expanding treatment options.

Those respondents initially attracted to surgery found that it is "too impersonal and divorced from the one-to-one contact I want" and involves "the same work every day." Specialties that do not offer direct patient care—pathology, radiology, or technical/evaluative fields—are not appealing to psychiatrists.

What Do You Like Most About Psychiatry?

Intellectual challenge brings the greatest enjoyment: "I like dealing with people's minds and the opportunity to use science and medicine as an applied method of helping people."

Satisfaction levels are reported to be lower than the total sample of physicians with 38.6 percent reporting themselves to be "very satisfied" and 22 percent "dissatisfied." There is a higher percentage (40.6 percent) of child psychiatrists responding, "very satisfied," and a lower percentage (19.8 percent) "dissatisfied." [6]

What Do You Like Least About Psychiatry?

The frustrations involve "inequities of reimbursement as compared to most other medical specialties," "the negative attitudes of the population to psychiatry and psychiatric patients," and "the legal aspects and dealing with courts." Marmor [7] offers the opinion that psychiatrists experience a "high degree of role strain" because of gaps between the public's expectations and reality, citing the fact that results of treatment are usually long-term with cures sometimes impossible to obtain. Also, when a treatment is successful, credit is given to the patient, denying the "ego-enhancing effects available to a surgeon whose operation has saved a life."

What Is Your Typical Daily Schedule?

Schedules and activities vary depending on the type of practice. A general psychiatrist will see patients in the hospital as well as in the office. Those on staff at a psychiatric hospital have a more structured schedule, often leading group sessions and working with multidisciplinary teams. A full-time administrator of a mental health center reports little clinical work and most time taken up by meetings and "politicking for funds."

Psychiatrists have on-call schedules for their own patients as well as for emergency rooms, but in general, they do not have to leave home very often at night or on weekends. Schedules seem to be less disruptive than in most other specialties.

What Abilities and Talents Are Important in Psychiatry?

The development of interpersonal skills is most important, both in establishing a doctor-patient relationship and in working with other health professionals. It is helpful to have "facility with language, both written and spoken," as well as the ability to listen.

What Personality Traits Best Characterize Psychiatrists?

As in surgery, a certain personality type is identified with psychiatry. They are often described as "the kinds of persons who have a question for everything that comes up."[8] Respondents see themselves as theoretic and analytic, but primarily as having a "sensitivity to others." They describe themselves as "calm" and "nonjudgmental," and as being content to interact with patients over a long period of time, often without seeing any results of their work.

The Myers-Briggs Type Indicator data report that general and child psychiatrists are similar in personality type, and that the field is attractive to people who focus on ideas, are interested in meanings and relationships, and who wish to understand rather than control events.

What Advice Would You Give a Medical Student Interested in Psychiatry?

Most respondents give guarded answers: "If you're interested, go for it. But understand that the clinical work is emotionally draining and the remuneration is low." One is more direct: "If you want money, go into surgery."

Specifically, you are advised to "learn to ask and expect answers to very personal topics: death, money, violence, etc. If you can do this and still relate to another person, then you have some ability to deal with the issues that affect others." In light of the increasingly scientific emphasis in psychiatry, you are advised to "get a good medical education, especially in cardiology, neurology, and endocrinology."

What Are the Future Challenges to Psychiatry?

"Psychiatry is still struggling to find its place in medicine," and "outcome studies will help put psychiatry on equal footing with other specialties." [2] However, scientific studies will be a challenge because there are hundreds of therapies to be evaluated.

Some respondents express concern about the "remedicalization" of psychiatry as a threat to the humanitarian side of the specialty, and others view the new focus on biochemistry and psychopharmacology as an opportunity to increase the status of the specialty.

New directions in psychiatry involve research on the brain, new medications for schizophrenia and substance abuse, and innovative treatments for depression.[9] One psychiatrist says, "Some of the advances occurring in this century will reveal how the mind and brain work. Because of that, it's the most exciting field in medicine." [10]

REFERENCES

1. Stone AA. The new paradox of psychiatric malpractice. *N Engl J Med* 1984; 311(21):1384–1387.
2. Lowes R. Psyched up, psyched out. *New Phys* 1995;44(10):23–27.
3. Szigethy E. Psychiatry's professional identity in the era of managed care. Resident forum. *JAMA* 1996;276(16):1284.

4. Lehrer DS, Kay J. Four decades of psychiatry. *Hosp Phys* 1997;33(9):11–15.
5. Weissman SH, Bashook PG. The 1982 first-year resident in psychiatry. *Am J Psychiatry* 1984;141(10):1240–1243.
6. Leigh JP, Kravitz RL, Schembri M, Samuels SJ, Mobley S. Physician career satisfaction across specialties. *Arch Intern Med* 2002; 162:1577-1584.
7. Marmor J. Psychiatrists may be prone to depression. *Am Med News* 1982;26(18):14.
8. Coombs RH. *Mastering medicine.* New York: The Free Press, 1978, pp. 196–198.
9. Barchas JD, Marzuk PM. General psychiatry. *JAMA* 1998;280(11):961–962.
10. Caserta M. Quoted by Fortson L. So you want to be a … *The New Physician* 2000; 49(6):31.

Job Values Selection of Psychiatrists

You can complete the questionnaires and obtain your scores for all specialties online at http://www.sdn.net, or compare your job values (as recorded in the Appendix) with the job values of psychiatrist respondents below:

Psychiatrists' Choices:	My Choices:
1. Working with people	1. _____
2. Working with my mind	2. _____
2. Achievement	3. _____
3. Independence	4. _____
(there is a tie for second place)	

No one chose: Working with my hands, good income, feedback from others.

Summary Profile of Psychiatrists   **My Personal Profile as a Psychiatrist**
(derived from questionnaire answers)

They tend to:	I tend to: (circle one number)				
	Never	Rarely	Sometimes	Frequently	Always
Ask why	1	2	3	4	5
Value independence highly	1	2	3	4	5
Have good listening skills/be interested in listening	1	2	3	4	5
Be adventurous/like challenges	1	2	3	4	5
Tolerate the unknown	1	2	3	4	5
Accept long-term outcomes	1	2	3	4	5
Be thinkers rather than "doers"	1	2	3	4	5
Be achievers	1	2	3	4	5
Be tolerant of others	1	2	3	4	5
Look for possibilities	1	2	3	4	5

Add total of numbers circled to get your TOTAL SCORE: _____

Transfer score to the Appendix.

Psychiatry

     sounds like me _____

     could be a possibility _____

     doesn't sound like me at all _____

Radiology

Diagnostic Radiology

FAST FACTS:

Number of first year residency positions offered in the NRMP in 2011: 144
Filled with US grads in 2011: 79.9%
Number of second year residency positions offered in the NRMP in 2011: 980
Filled with US grads in 2011: 78.9%
Length of training: 5 years, including a PGY-1 year
Number of residency programs: 193
Number of residents in training: 4,486
Competitiveness: High
Selection criteria for interview/ranking: USMLE scores, class rank, letters of recommendation
US senior matched applicants' mean Step 1 score: 238
US senior matched applicants' mean Step 2 score: 242
Number in US Board Certified in specialty: 19,094
Starting median compensation: $385,000
Median compensation for all physicians in specialty: $500,000
Average work hours per week: 58

THE DIAGNOSTIC RADIOLOGIST IS CONCERNED WITH THE application of x-rays and other forms of radiant energy to diagnose disease.

Residency Information. Residents train in diagnostic radiology for four years, usually after completing an internal medicine or surgery internship year. First-year and second-year positions are offered in diagnostic radiology through the National Resident Matching Program. Competitive applicants have membership in AOA, high grades, research and an elective in radiology.

There are one- to two-year fellowships in endovascular surgical neuroradiology, musculoskeletal, neuroradiology, abdominal, pediatric, cardiothoriacic and vascular/interventional radiology. There are also combined programs in diagnostic-nuclear radiology.

Board Certification. The American Board of Radiology awards certification in diagnostic radiology, radiation oncology, and radiation physics. The subspecialties are hospice and palliative care medicine, neuroradiology, nuclear radiology, pediatric radiology, and vascular and interventional radiology.

Supply and Projections. The recent large surplus of physicians in all areas of radiology has turned into a shortage for the following reasons: a drastic decline in the number of residents in the mid-1990s, an increase in the number of radiologists who retired at an earlier than expected age, and the demand for radiology services due to new imaging technology and an aging population. [1] However, "X-ray supertechnicians" are trained to do the work of a radiologist at a much lower cost. Also, new computer and technological advances may eventually reduce the need for radiologists. One radiologist cites the example of x-ray studies performed in Florida being read via teleradiology by radiologists in California.[2]

Even though half the medical students are women, only 28% of the radiology residents are women. It might be assumed that women desire more direct patient contact than men or view physics negatively. However, according to a recent survey of medical students,[3] the only deterrent cited by more women than men was the competitiveness of getting a radiology residency.

Economic Status and Types of Practice. Diagnostic radiologists' income is at the top levels. As hospital-based specialists, diagnostic radiologists have relatively low practice expenses because the hospital provides personnel, facilities, equipment, and supplies. In addition, this specialty employs nonphysicians to perform many services, thereby yielding a higher volume of patient care. Finally, reimbursement for services is often made by third-party payers who provide greater coverage for hospital services than for those offered in the office.

Traditionally, groups of radiologists contracted with hospitals to provide services for a negotiated amount of money. Newly graduated physicians have found themselves assigned to shift work as the specialty has become a 24 hour service in hospitals.

Further Information. The American College of Radiology, 1891 Preston White Drive, Reston, VA 22091. Telephone: (703) 648-8900 or (800) 227-5463. Internet address: www.acr.org.

A COMPOSITE PICTURE OF THE DIAGNOSTIC RADIOLOGIST

Why Choose Diagnostic Radiology?

Respondents report that they were attracted to radiology by its "cerebral nature," the "reasonably regular hours," and the new technologies. They report that they would not want to practice in fields that require taking care of chronically ill patients: "I liked the diagnostic aspects of cardiology, but disliked the care of chronic cardiac problems"; "I enjoy the diagnosis of perplexing problems, not the management of chronic, debilitating disease." Pathology was interesting to some, but "there was not enough contact with consulting physicians." Family medicine, internal medicine, and psychiatry are all characterized as having "too many gray areas" and not as challenging as radiology.

What Do You Like Most About Diagnostic Radiology?

Those radiologists who do more diagnostic work primarily enjoy the intellectual challenges and the "excitement of new technologies."

What Do You Like Least About Diagnostic Radiology?

Satisfaction levels are rising due to the recent increases in salary in response to a shortage of radiologists.

Other physicians are sometimes a source of stress: "overuse of x-rays by clinicians" and "clinicians who feel radiologists are not doctors, but technicians, and who resist my consultant role." Adequate clinical information may not be provided, further frustrating the radiologist. Blank[4] advocates two-way communication between primary care physicians and radiologists, validating the respondents' complaints.

What Is Your Typical Daily Schedule?

Although each day of the week may be different, there tends to be a similar weekly schedule. Certain tests and procedures are performed only on certain days in some hospitals; others are done daily. Depending upon the setting, diagnostic radiologists report dividing their time between computed tomography (CT), ultrasound, and magnetic resonance imaging (MRI) procedures, as well as more general x-rays. A few hours each day are spent reviewing x-ray films and consulting with referring physicians.

Some respondents report being on-call for emergencies, but for considerably less time than most other specialties.

What Abilities and Talents Are Important in Diagnostic Radiology?

Interpersonal skills are needed in diagnostic radiology to deal with physician and technologist colleagues.

Technological and mathematical skills, as well as a "broad base of pathologic and anatomic knowledge," are necessary. You need the "ability to master spatial relationships in three dimensions, above average visual acuity," and good hand-eye coordination.

What Personality Traits Best Characterize Diagnostic Radiologists?

Radiologists describe themselves as "intellectually curious," "relaxed and slightly eccentric," and "not too uptight." The Myers-Briggs Type Indicator data[5] report that radiologists are significantly more analytical and perceptive than other physicians.

What Advice Would You Give a Medical Student Interested in Diagnostic Radiology?

Students are advised to spend time learning about the variety of choices in radiology. Respondents all agree that this is a rapidly changing field, suitable for an individual interested in diagnosis and technology. One respondent specifically says, "The more anatomy learned, the better."

An elective in radiology, research in the field, and a strong background in clinical medicine are all advised.

What Are the Future Challenges to Diagnostic Radiology?

All respondents cite the task of keeping up with the rapidly developing technologies in radiology. Evens[5] feels that there is "no end in sight" and describes the development of electronic radiography and the acceptance of mammography and MRI. Technologies in the subspecialty of interventional radiology fuel its rapid growth, as in the treatment of aortic aneurysms.[7] There is, however, at least in the opinion of one respondent, the need to "not let medicine become too mechanized and overshadow the reason for our being, i.e., the patient."

There are continuing questions concerning the future direction of subspecialization within radiology. Some believe that radiology should be system oriented and some advocate technique orientation. As diagnostic radiology began to subspecialize it was primarily into system divisions, such as gastrointestinal, nervous, and respiratory systems. Today there are fellowship programs established along both organ system and technology lines, e.g., in gastroenterologic radiology and neuroradiology, but also in sonography and computed tomography. Seen as still being in a developmental stage, radiology's own internal structure and role in patient care are discussed and debated.

Finally, the influence of insurance companies on how radiology studies are ordered and performed is a considerable challenge. There are turf battles over who is qualified to interpret images[8] because Medicare and third-party payers are unwilling to pay for more than one person interpreting the image.

REFERENCES

1. Compensation Monitor. Radiologists, anesthesiologists in demand. Managed Care 2002; 11(4):25.
2. Bichel JC. Radiology and dinosaurs. *Unique Opportunities* 1997;7(4):60–64.
3. Fielding JR et al. Choosing a specialty in medicine:female medical students and radiology. Amer Jour Rad 2007;188:897-900.
4. Blank P. Do you really need to order that radiograph? *Phys Management* 1998; 38(1):29–30.
5. McCaulley MH. Application of the Myers-Briggs Type Indicator to medicine and other health professions, Monograph I. Gainesville, FL: Center for Applications of Psychological Type, Inc., 1978, pp. 253–254.
6. Evens RG. Radiology. *JAMA* 1991;265(23):3167–3168.
7. Evens RG. Radiology. *JAMA* 1997;277(23):1897–1898.
8. Tilke B. Radiologists ask: Who's reading medical images? *Amer Med News* 1998; 41(31):24–25.

Job Values of Diagnostic Radiologists

You can complete the questionnaires and obtain your scores for all specialties online at http://www.sdn.net, or compare your job values (as recorded in the Appendix) with the job values of diagnostic radiologist respondents below:

Diagnostic Radiologists' Choices:	My Choices:
1. Independence	1. _____
2. Sufficient time off	2. _____
2. Working with my mind	3. _____
2. Creativity	4. _____
(there is a three-way tie for second place)	

No one chose: Variety, good income, security, prestige, taking care of people, feedback from others

Summary Profile of Diagnostic Radiologists (derived from questionnaire answers)	My Personal Profile as a Diagnostic Radiologist				
They tend to:	I tend to: (circle one number)				
	Never	Rarely	Sometimes	Frequently	Always
Value time off	1	2	3	4	5
Like complex problem solving	1	2	3	4	5
Value independence highly	1	2	3	4	5
Enjoy being an "expert"	1	2	3	4	5
Be easy going	1	2	3	4	5
Have interests outside of medicine	1	2	3	4	5
Be adventurous/like challenges	1	2	3	4	5
Be uncomfortable with poorly defined problems	1	2	3	4	5
Think logically	1	2	3	4	5
Be visually oriented	1	2	3	4	5

Add total of numbers circled to get your TOTAL SCORE: _____

Transfer score to the Appendix.

Diagnostic radiology

sounds like me _____

could be a possibility _____

doesn't sound like me at all _____

Radiation Oncology

FAST FACTS:

Number of first year residency positions offered in the NRMP in 2011: 16

Filled with US grads in 2011: 93.8%

Number of second year residency positions offered in the NRMP in 2011: 155

Filled with US grads in 2011: 96.8%

Length of training: 5 years, including a PGY-1 year

Number of residency programs: 83

Number of residents in training: 608

Competitiveness: Very High

Selection criteria for interview/ranking: grade in elective in the specialty, number of honors grades, published medical school research, grades in required clerkships, a strong background in physics

US senior matched applicants' mean Step 1 score: 238

US senior matched applicants' mean Step 2 score: 241

Number in US Board Certified in specialty: 3,414

Median compensation for all physicians in specialty: $375,000

Average work hours per week: 56

EVEN THOUGH THE AMERICAN BOARD OF RADIOLOGY REC-ognized therapeutic radiology (now called radiation oncology) as a distinct field as early as 1934, initially it was practiced mostly by surgeons or as "a sideline to radiodiagnosis."[1] The radiation oncologist treats the patient with x-rays, radium, and radionuclides. As a clinical practice, the "art of working with cancer patients" is as important as "the physical and biologic underpinnings of this interesting field."[2]

Residency Information. Applicants need to complete a transitional or preliminary internship year before starting their radiation oncology training. Competitive applicants also have a strong background in physics and research interest. The residency curriculum includes rotations through oncology subspecialties to provide a broad understanding of oncology.

Board Certification. The American Board of Radiology awards board certification in radiation oncology. You need to pass both written and oral examinations.

Supply and Projections. An American College of Radiology survey[3] of 600 radiology groups revealed that there was a serious shortage of employment opportunities as recent as eight years ago; but, the situation is rapidly changing. Demand for radiation therapy is expected to grow 10 times faster than supply between 2010 and 2020. [3]

Economic Status and Types of Practice. Radiation oncologists earn above the average income of US physicians. As hospital-based specialists, radiation oncologists have relatively low practice expenses because the hospital provides personnel, facilities, equipment, and supplies. In addition, this specialty employs non-physicians to perform many services, thereby yielding a higher volume of patient care. Finally, reimbursement for services is often made by third-party payers who provide greater coverage for hospital services than for those offered in the office.

Further Information. The American Society for Radiology Oncology, 8280 Willow Oaks Corporate Drive, Suite 500, Fairfax, VA 22031. Telephone (703)502-1550. Internet address: www.astro.org.

A COMPOSITE PICTURE OF THE RADIATION ONCOLOGIST

Why Choose Radiation Oncology?

Medical schools do not offer radiation oncology as a required part of the curriculum, and therefore it is often chosen on the basis of less actual experience than some of the other specialties. Respondents report that they were attracted to radiation oncology by the "reasonably regular hours" and the new technologies. Some found the intense patient relationship that may last beyond the expected four to six weeks of treatment to be an initial attraction.

What Do You Like Most About Radiation Oncology?

"The feeling that I can intervene and perhaps cure someone is very satisfying." All respondents enjoy procedures requiring manual dexterity, skill, and experience. Also liked are the interactions with clinical physicians, time off, and the consultant role.

What Do You Like Least About Radiation Oncology?

"It is difficult to form relationships with patients and then see them die." This theme is similar to the views expressed by medical oncologists.

What Is Your Typical Daily Schedule?

Radiation oncologists work in hospital settings and have a predictable patient care schedule. In academic centers, more time is spent on research and teaching than in community hospitals. There is little night call.

What Abilities and Talents Are Important in Radiation Oncology?

Communication skills are needed to effectively deal with seriously ill cancer patients and their family members. In addition, radiation oncologists work with radiation technologists and must be able to work on a team.

What Personality Traits Best Characterize Radiation Oncologists?

Radiation oncologists describe themselves as "compassionate." Myers-Briggs Type Indicator studies[4] indicate that radiation oncology seems to attract those who enjoy patient care.

What Advice Would You Give a Medical Student Interested in Radiation Oncology?

"Learn as much as possible about anatomy, surgical oncology, and chemotherapy during medical school and internship." An interest in research is valued at larger residency programs. Also, a strong background in physics is "helpful."

What Are the Future Challenges to Radiation Oncology?

All respondents cite the task of keeping up with radiobiologic concepts. There also are pressures to give greater consideration to patients' quality-of-life despite the difficulty of measuring this subjective variable.[2]

REFERENCES

1. del Regato JA, Brady LW. Therapeutic radiology. *JAMA* 1981;245:2222.
2. Gunn W. Book review: Principles and practice of radiation oncology. *JAMA* 1998; 279(17):1406.
3. Smith BD, Haffty BG, Wilson, LD et al. The future of radiation oncology in the United States from 2010 to 2020: will supply keep pace with demand? J Clin Oncol 2010 Dec 10; 28(35):5160-5165.
4. Bushee GR, Sunshine JH, Chan WC, Shaffer KA. The demand side of the job market for diagnostic radiologists and radiation oncologists: Hiring by physician groups in 1995. *Am J Roentgenol* 1996;167(2):303–309.
5. McCaulley MH. Application of the Myers-Briggs Type Indicator to medicine and other health professions, Monograph I. Gainesville, FL: Center for Applications of Psychological Type, Inc., 1978, pp. 253–254.

Job Values Selection of Radiation Oncologists

You can complete the questionnaires and obtain your scores for all specialties online at http://www.sdn.net, or compare your job values (as recorded in the Appendix) with the job values of radiation oncologist respondents below:

Radiation Oncologists' Choices:	My Choices:
1. Taking care of people	1. _____
2. Decision making	2. _____
3. Working with my hands	3. _____
4. Sufficient time off	4. _____

They tend to:	I tend to: (circle one number)				
Summary Profile of Radiation Oncologists (derived from questionnaire answers)	My Personal Profile as a Radiation Oncologist				
	Never	Rarely	Sometimes	Frequently	Always
Enjoy taking care of people	1	2	3	4	5
Enjoy being an "expert"	1	2	3	4	5
Have manual dexterity	1	2	3	4	5
Be team players	1	2	3	4	5
Prefer a planned schedule	1	2	3	4	5
Act decisively	1	2	3	4	5
Have good listening skills/ interested in listening	1	2	3	4	5
Accept long-term outcomes	1	2	3	4	5
Be comfortable with their own mortality	1	2	3	4	5
Be optimistic	1	2	3	4	5

Add total of numbers circled to get your TOTAL SCORE: _____

Transfer score to the Appendix.

Radiation oncology

sounds like me _____

could be a possibility _____

doesn't sound like me at all _____

Surgery, General

GENERAL SURGERY IS THE BASIC DISCIPLINE FROM WHICH other surgical subspecialties have emerged. Dr. James B. Snow, an otolaryngologist, addressing the 1983 Congress of the American College of Surgeons, said, "All of surgery depends on the discipline of general surgery for fundamental research in perioperative care, wound healing and nutrition."[1]

Surgery, by definition, deals with diseases or injuries that require operative procedures. Because of the life-and-death nature of many situations a surgeon confronts, there is an aura of magic and power surrounding this specialty. Medical school students have opportunities to observe surgeons at work and often decide about the suitability of this specialty for their own individual talents and personalities.

Residency Information. A general surgery residency requires five years of training. You can apply for a "categorical" internship—the beginning year of a general surgery training program—and be assured that if you successfully complete the first year, you can continue for four more years in the same program. Or you may prefer a "preliminary" program in which positions are available for one or two years, but there is no assurance that you will be able to complete the full five years at that institution. There is usually less competition for the latter program and it may be the right choice for those who wish to enter a surgical subspecialty.

There are a number of pathways, from 5 to 7 years, to train in vascular surgery. In 2011 27 programs offered 30 first year positions and these were filled by 96.7% US grads, making this one of the most competitive fields for a first year residency. You can match to a integrated vascular surgery 5 year residency program directly from medical school or you can be in an "independent pathway" with 3-5 years of surgery followed by 2-3 years of vascular surgery training. Also available after residency are one- or two-year fellowships in trauma surgery. You need to negotiate with programs on an individual basis for these fellowships.

Board Certification. Five years of training beyond medical school and successful completion of extensive written, oral, and clinical testing are prerequisites for board certification.

Specialized training and certification are available in pediatric surgery, vascular surgery, hand surgery, hospice and palliative care and surgical critical care. This training is distinguished from those surgical areas with separate primary boards (colon and rectal surgery, neurological surgery, obstetrics-gynecology, ophthalmology, orthopaedic surgery, otolaryngology, plastic surgery, thoracic surgery, and urology), each discussed in separate chapters in this book.

Supply and Projections. The surgical profession's own workforce studies[2] have been indicating a shortage of general surgeons, especially in rural areas. The number of applicants to general surgery residency programs has fallen 30 percent in the past 10 years.[3] Bland and Isaacs[4] cite lifestyle issues as a major factor in a student's decision not to become a general surgeon. A survey of vascular surgeons[5] also reports a potential shortage in this field. Growth in the numbers of pediatric generalist surgeons reached a plateau by 2006, while there was a 24 percent increase in pediatric surgical subspecialists.[6]

Economic Status and Types of Practice. Income levels reflect geographic needs, but general surgeons are paid less than surgical subspecialists. A surgeon delayed in the operating room is often paying employees who wait in the office for his or her arrival. Similarly, costly office equipment is not used fully because surgeon time is divided between the hospital and office. There is concern that private practice is diminishing and that hospital-employed surgery is increasing.[7]

A general surgeon can practice in a solo or group practice, in an urban or rural setting, or in an academic or research institution. Third-world countries need surgeons, for either short- or long-term commitments.

Further Information. The American College of Surgeons, 633 N. St. Clair Street, Chicago, IL 60611. Telephone: (312) 202-5000. Internet address: www.facs.org. I also recommend the booklet "So You Want To Be A Surgeon . . ." by David M. Heimbach, M.D. and Kaj Johansen, M.D., Department of Surgery, University of Washington School of Medicine, Seattle, WA 98104.

A COMPOSITE PICTURE OF THE GENERAL SURGEON

Why Choose General Surgery?

All respondents decided to be a surgeon very early in their careers, some even prior to medical school, and many were influenced by "authorities within the medical school." There seems to be an attempt by medical students to assess themselves in relationship to surgeons: "much of what seemed to be required in excelling in surgery was present in my personality and outlook."

In choosing this specialty one respondent was aware that, "As a *general* surgeon, one needs to still remain a well-rounded physician with a broad approach to patients." However, surgeons report that internal medicine is not appealing because it is "intangible," has a "lack of variety in patient care and daily routine," and involves "chronic problems." Radiology and pathology have "too little patient contact." In psychiatry and neurology a physician can "rarely cure disease." Most respondents only ever considered being surgeons. "I never wanted to be anything except a surgeon!"

What Do You Like Most About General Surgery?

There is unanimous agreement that general surgeons enjoy being in the operating room "making patients well by doing something active." There is "a sense of involvement in changing the course of a disease."

"I enjoy two things very much. One is the close relationship I have with my patients and their gratitude when they come through a difficult surgery with good results. I also enjoy the technical problems at the time of surgery and the satisfaction of solving these problems."

The "very satisfied" percentage (43 percent) is slightly higher than that of all physicians (42.3 percent) in the survey, but the percentage (20.4 percent) of those dissatisfied is higher than than the total (17.6 percent). [8]

What Do You Like Least About General Surgery?

Complaints about "charts and paperwork," "bureaucracy," "the politics of academics," and "the business aspects of private practice" all reflect the surgeon's dislike of nonaction-oriented activities.

The long hours and dealing with dying patients are also described as unpleasant aspects of the specialty.

What Is Your Typical Daily Schedule?

AMA statistics report that surgeons practice an average of 60 hours per week, and respondents report working 10- to 12-hour weekdays plus night and weekend duties. "Except when out of town, I go to the hospital at least daily without fail."

A typical day begins about 7:00 AM with hospital rounds on pre- and post-operative patients. This is followed by approximately three to four hours of surgery (one to three operative cases per day), three hours in the office seeing patients, and another hour in the hospital making rounds or consulting. In addition, there are medical staff meetings, teaching conferences, and administrative tasks each day. Some surgeons are on call all the time; others share a coverage schedule with colleagues. Many in private practice are scheduled for hospital emergency room call in addition to private practice patients.

A general surgeon's practice is semi-emergency in nature, and operations may be performed at all hours. There are various problems—appendicitis, hernia, gall bladder disease, ulcer disease, bowel obstruction—which are related to the abdomen. General surgeons do a considerable amount of minor surgery—nevi, abscesses, cysts—and manage some nonsurgical conditions such as thrombophlebitis. One respondent enjoys electrophysiology and pacemakers; another is director of a burn center. A pediatric surgeon's practice deals with congenital anomalies, cancer, and trauma; the vascular surgeons focus on arterial reconstructive operations.

What Abilities and Talents Are Important in General Surgery?

"An ability and willingness to work hard and for extended periods of time; the capability to think, decide, and act quickly; manual skill and dexterity; and the ability to recall a large volume of information needed to cover the specialty of general surgery."

What Personality Traits Best Characterize General Surgeons?

Of all the specialties, surgery is probably the most identified with a "personality type." General surgeons report themselves to be decisive, aggressive, "doers not talkers," compulsive, perfectionistic, and hard working.

However, McCaulley [9] has identified differences in individuals choosing surgical specialties—some resemble each other closely and others do not. General surgeons are thought to be more similar in personality type to those choosing obstetrics, ophthalmology, ortho-paedic surgery, and urology, who prefer dealing with problems in a straightforward manner by direct action than to those selecting plastic, neurological, and thoracic surgery, who prefer dealing with complex and subtle problems.

What Advice Would You Give a Medical Student Interested in General Surgery?

All respondents advise the medical student interested in surgery to prepare for a lifestyle that involves long hours and requires an under-standing partner and family. One says, "Be sure you fit." And another advises, "If you can find anything else you would be happy doing, *DO THAT* rather than general surgery. If you can find nothing else that has the same aura, magic, appeal, and attraction, then come on in."

Students are encouraged to attend department conferences and to get to know individual surgeons on the faculty.

What Are the Future Challenges to General Surgery?

The major challenge is to prevent the continuing decline in medical students choosing to train as general surgeons in the face of an aging population. Meeting the challenge of the mandate of an 80- hour work week for all residents required use of new technologies for teaching such as the computer generated "virtual" surgical expe-rience and the hiring of more support staff to do tasks previously performed by residents. [3] There is still controversy over the benefits of the 80 hour work week. [10]

Although there is a strong call for an effort to prevent further fragmentation of general surgery, most feel that there are many challenges within general surgery itself: "Reconstructive surgery and organ replacement are only in their infancy," "surgery with lasers," "surgery on the unborn child." On the other hand, there is a warning that surgeons need to "maintain involvement with the patient rather than with technology."

There is a call for a collaborative multispecialty approach with interventional radiologists and other interventionalists in the use of endovascular technologies to minimize costs and turf battles.[11] Another challenge is whether vascular surgery should have a separate board and residency review committee.[12]

REFERENCES

1. Snow JB. Quoted in: Carey LC. Surgery in transition. *Postgrad Med* 1984;75(1):13–19.

2. Lynge DC, Larson EH, Thompson MJ et al. A longitudinal analysis of the general surgery workforce in the United States, 1981-2005. *Arch Surg*; 2008 Apr; 143(4):345-350.

3. Hurt A. Where have all the surgeons gone? *The New Physician* 2002; 51(7):28-33.

4. Bland KI, Isaacs G. Contemporary trends in student selection of medical specialties. Archives of Surgery 2002; 137(3)

5. Satiani B, Williams TE, Go MR. Predicted shortage of vascular surgeons in the United States: population and workload analysis. *J Vasc Surg; 2009 Oct; 50(4):946-952.*

6. Poley S, Ricketts T, Belsky D, Gaul K. Pediatric surgeons: subspecialists increase faster than generalists. Bull Amer Coll Surg 2010; 95(10):35-38.

7. Swanson RS. Governors' Committee on Surgical Practice: An update. Bull Amer Coll Surg 2010; 95(10):29-30.

8. Leigh JP, Kravitz RL, Schembri M, Samuels SJ, Mobley S. Physician career satisfaction across specialties. *Arch Intern Med* 2002; 162:1577-1584.

9. McCaulley MH. Application of the Myers-Briggs Type Indicator to medicine and other health professions, Monograph I.

Gainesville, FL: Center for Applications of Psychological Type. 1978, p. 239, 236.

10. Dehmer JJ. Young Dinosaurs fighting extinction. Arc Surg 2010; 145(11):1037-1038.

11. Veith FJ, Marin ML. Endovascular technology and its impact on the relationship among vascular surgeons, interventional radiologists and other specialists. *World J Surg* 1996;20(6):687–691.

12. Veith FJ. Leaving the nest: Should vascular surgery seek board status separate from general surgery? *Semin Vasc Surg* 1997;10(2):81–84.

General Surgeons' Choices

You can complete the questionnaires and obtain your scores for all specialties online at http://www.sdn.net, or compare your job values (as recorded in the Appendix) with the job values of general surgeon respondents below:

General Surgeons' Choices	My Choices:
1. Decision making	1. _____
2. Taking care of people	2. _____
2. Variety	3. _____
3. Independence	4. _____
3. Achievement	
(there are ties for second and third place)	

No one chose: Security, prestige, sufficient time off, feedback from others.

Summary Profile of General Surgeons (derived from questionnaire answers)	My Personal Profile as a General Surgeon				
They tend to:	I tend to: (circle one number)				
	Never	Rarely	Sometimes	Frequently	Always
Enjoy taking care of people	1	2	3	4	5
Value independence highly	1	2	3	4	5
Have manual dexterity	1	2	3	4	5
Need to see tangible results of their efforts quickly	1	2	3	4	5
Act decisively	1	2	3	4	5
Be achievers	1	2	3	4	5
Identify with role models	1	2	3	4	5
Be "doers" rather than talkers	1	2	3	4	5
Deal with problems straight-forwardly with direct action	1	2	3	4	5
Be perfectionistic	1	2	3	4	5

Add total of numbers circled to get your TOTAL SCORE:_____

Transfer score to the Appendix.

General surgery

sounds like me_____

could be a possibility_____

doesn't sound like me at all_____

Thoracic Surgery

THE COMPLEX ETHICAL AND LEGAL ASPECTS OF HEART SURGERY that arose from technological advances in thoracic surgery have made society acutely aware of this field. Thoracic surgery (also called "cardiothoracic surgery" and "cardiovascular and thoracic surgery") deals with surgery of the chest cavity containing the heart, lungs, and esophagus.

Residency Information. Thoracic surgery has traditionally required the longest period of residency training—a minimum of five years of general surgery followed by two years of a fellowship in thoracic surgery. Almost everyone applies for a residency position in thoracic surgery through the National Resident Matching Program Specialties Matching Service when you are in the second or third year of your general surgery training.

The only way a fourth year medical student can apply is through the NRMP for the Integrated Pathway. The direct track residency is six years in length and in 2010 there were 10 positions offered in 10 programs with an 80 percent US graduates' match rate.

There is a one year fellowship in congenital cardiac surgery following completion of the residency in thoracic surgery that is offered in 10 programs.

The two year osteopathic programs begin after three years of general surgery and one year of internship.

Board Certification. Certification by the American Board of Surgery is a prerequisite to examination by the American Board of Thoracic Surgery. In addition, two years of residency training in thoracic and cardiovascular surgery are required to take the separate written and oral examinations.

Supply and Projections. The number of physicians in this specialty is projected to decrease 21 percent by 2020 because the number training in this specialty is too low to replace the number who will retire. [1] Cited as factors are lifestyle issues, high professional liability risks, and long years of training.

Economic Status and Types of Practice. Thoracic surgeons' incomes are in the highest ranges of surgical subspecialists. Thoracic surgeons practice in urban areas because they need a large population base to support their practices.

Further Information. The Society of Thoracic Surgeons, 633 N. Saint Clair Street, Suite 2320, Chicago, IL 60611. Telephone: (312)202-5800. Internet address: www.sts.org.

A COMPOSITE PICTURE OF THE THORACIC SURGEON

Why Choose Thoracic Surgery?

The personal contact with a thoracic surgeon during medical school was a significant factor in specialty choice for many respondents: "I decided to enter cardiothoracic surgery following my second year of medical school. I was offered a position working in the laboratory of a cardiothoracic surgeon. His personality and the exposure to the nature and content of the cardiothoracic subspecialty strongly influenced my selection," and "The opportunity of working with a cardiac surgeon during an externship program between the junior and senior years of medical school was the deciding factor."

Respondents were attracted to the field by the opportunity to help critically ill patients "whose life depended directly on the outcome of the surgery." They all say that they would not want to practice in a specialty that involved the continuing care of chronically ill patients. A significant number were attracted to plastic surgery, but rejected it because it did not afford the opportunity to correct life-threatening conditions. However, both the appeal and the opportunity were found in thoracic surgery: "technical demands of the operation require good technique to get a good result."

What Do You Like Most About Thoracic Surgery?

A good outcome from surgery is the major satisfaction of this specialty. "In the majority of cases, successful surgery allows a complete rehabilitation, often within a very short period of time. The gratitude and respect derived from the patient as a result of this are enormous."

More than half of the physicians surveyed report that they are "very satisfied (53.4 percent) with 17.8 percent, "dissatisfied." [2]

What Do You Like Least About Thoracic Surgery?

The answers are chiefly related to patient care: "The least enjoyable aspects are the complications and the occasional deaths which result from attempted operations and the pain of communicating with the families about the catastrophe which may have occurred," and "The most difficult task in my situation is the allocation of my most valuable resource, time. It often seems as if demands are being made from all sides regarding the use of one's time."

What Is Your Typical Daily Schedule?

The average 12-hour work day is spent primarily in the hospital making rounds and performing operations that can last for many hours. Occasionally emergency operations will involve evening hours. The thoracic surgeon is also on call for his or her postoperative patients, in addition to any other call arrangements made with colleagues. There is frequent communication by telephone with nurses who are caring for critically ill patients. The patient population is usually older adults, with an average age of 55 to 60.

What Abilities and Talents Are Important in Thoracic Surgery?

There is a strong intellectual and scientific bent in many practitioners of cardiothoracic surgery. It is also necessary to master the technical skills and a "relatively well-developed hand-eye coordination although I believe this skill can be learned by anyone diligent enough to practice the technique involved."

A thoracic surgeon needs "to think logically and in a step-wise fashion to arrive at the correct decisions before, during, and after the operative procedure."

One respondent says, "The most important ability is to be able to enforce calmness in the face of an impending catastrophe."

What Personality Traits Best Characterize Thoracic Surgeons?

"Compulsive, hard-working, and highly motivated individuals" are found in this specialty. They are described as being "self-assured" and able to motivate and direct subordinates.

The Myers-Briggs Type Indicator data show thoracic surgeons to be more similar in personality type to neurological and plastic surgeons than to other surgeons. They are described as being action oriented, concerned with possibilities, decisive, and well-organized.

What Advice Would You Give a Medical Student Interested in Thoracic Surgery?

"I would recommend that a student interested in this specialty spend elective time in the laboratory or on the ward with a thoracic surgeon. Should interest be further aroused, I would advise completing a general surgical residency in the same institution in which one wishes to pursue a thoracic residency. This is, however, not mandatory." Residents in general surgery who are planning to take a year of training in a laboratory setting are advised to choose a cardiovascular surgical facility.

What Are the Future Challenges to Thoracic Surgery?

The trend is for physicians in this specialty to focus their practices on either cardiothoracic or thoracic surgery exclusively. There are an increased number of adult congenital cardiac patients.[3]

One respondent says, "The development of nonsurgical methods of treating coronary artery disease such as balloon dilatation, laser catheterizations, etc., may somewhat limit any growth in this specialty. Conversely, if a satisfactory artificial heart which is totally implantable can be developed, the number of cardiac operations may increase."

REFERENCES

1. Grover A, Gorman K, Dall TM et al. Shortage of cardiothoracic surgeons is likely by 2020. *Circulation*; 2009 August 11; 120(6):488-494.
2. Leigh JP, Kravitz RL, Schembri M, Samuels SJ, Mobley S. Physician career satisfaction across specialties. *Arch Intern Med;* 2002; 162:1577-1584.
3. Slater M. Oregon Health & Science University, Portland, Oregon. Personal communication, January 27, 2011.

Job Values Selection of Thoracic Surgeons

You can complete the questionnaires and obtain your scores for all specialties online at http://www.sdn.net, or compare your job values (as recorded in the Appendix) with the job values of thoracic surgeon respondents below:

Thoracic Surgeons' Choices:	My Choices:
1. Creativity	1. _____
1. Decision making	2. _____
2. Working with my hands	3. _____
3. Working with my mind	4. _____
(there is a tie for first place)	

No one chose: Sufficient time off, feedback from others.

Summary Profile of Thoracic Surgeons (derived from questionnaire answers)	**My Personal Profile as a Thoracic Surgeon**				
They tend to:	I tend to: (circle one number)				
	Never	Rarely	Sometimes	Frequently	Always
Like complex problem solving	1	2	3	4	5
Have manual dexterity	1	2	3	4	5
Need to see tangible results of their efforts quickly	1	2	3	4	5
Act decisively	1	2	3	4	5
Be adventurous/like challenges	1	2	3	4	5
Be a leader	1	2	3	4	5
Be energetic/have a high energy level	1	2	3	4	5
Think logically	1	2	3	4	5
Be perfectionistic	1	2	3	4	5
Look for possibilities	1	2	3	4	5

Add total of numbers circled to get your TOTAL SCORE:_____

Transfer score to the Appendix.

Thoracic surgery

    sounds like me _____

    could be a possibility _____

    doesn't sound like me at all _____

Urology

FAST FACTS:

Number of first year residency positions offered in the NRMP in 2010: 9 (most positions are offered through the AUA Urology Matching Program)

Number of advanced year positions offered in 2010 in the AUA Match: 268

Filled with US grads in 2010: 88%

Length of training: 5 years, including a minimum PGY-1 year in general surgery

Number of residency programs: 114

Number of residents in training: 969

Competitiveness: Very high

Selection criteria for interview/ranking: USMLE scores, AOA membership, honors in a urology elective, letters of recommendation from urologists, research, inquisitive nature, manual dexterity

Number in US Board Certified in specialty: 8,510

Starting median compensation: $190,000

Median compensation for all physicians in specialty: $276,798

Average work hours per week: 61

KARL MENNINGER[1] OBSERVED, "PERHAPS THE UROLOGISTS are the frankest and, in a sense, the most unrepressed of all the specialists." He perceives them as being almost immune to conjectures regarding their motivations for choosing the specialty of urology, and judges them to be "unusually open-minded."

Urology is a surgical subspecialty concerned with the medical and surgical treatment of disorders and diseases of the female urinary tract and male urogenital tract. Urologists are involved with problems of the kidney, ureters, bladder, prostate, urethra, and male genital structure. Often the urologist and nephrologist coordinate their efforts in treating patients with kidney disease.

Residency Training. More than 200 residency positions are offered each year through the American Urology Association (AUA) Residency Match. You also need to register with the National Resident Matching Program (NRMP) for one or two years of training that are initially spent preferably in general surgery. This is followed by a minimum of three years of urology training.

Board Certification. Candidates must pass a written examination within three years of completing residency. A second oral examination must be taken within five years of successful completion of the first examination. Recertification is required after 10 years.

While there is no subspecialty certification offered in urology, guidelines have been established for special training programs in pediatric urology, renal transplantation, urologic oncology, and male and female reproductive surgery.

Supply and Projections. A workforce study[2] conducted by the American Urological Association reported that if graduate numbers remain stable, the future supply will be in balance with patient-care needs. However, concerns about prostate cancer and erectile dysfunction will increase as the population ages, potentially leading to more need for urologists.

Economic Status and Types of Practice. Incomes are less than some other surgical sub-specialties because of the amount of non-compensated counseling time offered. Most urologists are in private fee-for-service practice, usually in urban settings.

Further Information. The American Urological Association, 1000 Corporate Boulevard, Linthicum, Maryland 21090. Telephone: 866-746-4282. Internet address: www.auanet.org The website has extensive information for medical students about residency application and the urology match.

A COMPOSITE PICTURE OF THE UROLOGIST
Why Choose Urology?

Personal contact with urologists, either as friends or role models, was a strong factor in the respondents' specialty choice. One says, "I did renal research in medical school and had association with urologists during my internship." Another cites: "Various people—a surgeon during my internship, a friend in residency—led me to urology." The specific appeal is that urology offers "a broad scope of activities in a limited, fairly succinct specialty." Also, the combination of medical and surgical treatment, a wide range of patients, and clear outcomes of one's work are reported as reasons for choosing this specialty.

Other surgical specialties were considered, but "general surgery is being eroded by other specialties"; "cardiopulmonary surgery involves long operating hours and is high tension"; "obstetrics has bad hours"; and "orthopaedics has too many chronic care patients, legal cases, and emergency call." Respondents say they would not want to practice general medicine: "too broad in scope for me to feel comfortable knowing what I am doing" and "I like to operate, cure, and move to another problem."

What Do You Like Most About Urology?

Urologists enjoy operating most of all. Also satisfying is "working in a field in which one can be relatively certain of the disease process and its cause."

More urologists report themselves to be "very satisfied" (48%) and less "dissatisfied" (13.8%) than the total of physicians surveyed in one study. [3]

What Do You Like Least About Urology?

Urologists seem very satisfied with their specialty, offering only "paperwork" and "poorly motivated, demanding patients" as negatives, neither of which is unique to the specialty of urology.

What Is Your Typical Daily Schedule?

The length of a urologist's work day is reported to be less than other surgeons, with an average of 9 to 10 hours. The practice is a combination of surgery and office visits and involves caring for patients of all ages, from newborns to the elderly, usually referred by primary care physicians. On-call responsibilities vary with the type of practice and population served, but there is less emergency work than other surgical specialties, such as orthopaedic surgery.

What Abilities and Talents Are Important in Urology?

In addition to the surgical skills of manual dexterity and good eye-hand coordination, the urologist needs to develop counseling skills because many problems will have psychological aspects, especially those involving sexual problems. Problems with infertility, impotence, and genitourinary function require the physician to take time talking to patients. In addition, the urologist who performs kidney transplantations must deal with the ethical dilemmas concerning scarce resources.

What Personality Traits Best Characterize Urologists?

Many respondents see themselves as "outgoing." They like to have people around and it is easy for them to communicate freely. Typically, they are interested in the results of their work, and dislike long, slow activities. They particularly like to work in a fairly limited specialty so they can feel comfortable in learning the necessary skills.

What Advice Would You Give a Medical Student Interested in Urology?

Students are advised to start planning early—do an elective in urology, make good grades, and get good surgical experience.

One respondent advises students to assess if they enjoy urology enough to: "devote time to prolonged education; and all things considered, make less money than you might in another specialty."

What Are the Future Challenges to Urology?

The technological changes have some stressful aspects: "High-tech machinery may eliminate many operations we presently do," and "We need to adjust to the rapidly changing surgical technique advances."

The challenge of the previously small number of women urologists at a time when womens' urologic conditions, such as incontinence and infections, are increasing[4] has been taken seriously. With the increasing number of women selecting urology as their specialty choice, a recent survey[5] of female urology residents documents the challenge of negative behavior by male patients and male colleagues.

REFERENCES

1. Menninger K. Psychological factors in the choice of medicine as a profession. *Bulletin of the Menninger Clinic* 1957;21:100.
2. McCullough DL. Manpower needs in urology in the twenty-first century. *Urol Clin N Am* 1998;25(1):15–22.
3. Leigh JP, Kravitz RL, Schembri M, Samuels SJ, Mobley S. Physician career satisfaction across specialties. *Arch Intern Med* 2002; 162:1577-1584.
4. Katola SJ. Rites of passage. *Life in Medicine* 1996;5(1):32–36.
5. Jackson I, Bobbin M, Jordan M, Baker S. A survey of women urology residents regarding career choice and practice challenges. *J Womens Health (Larchmt)*;2009 Nov;18(11):1867 1872.

Job Values Selection of Urologists

You can complete the questionnaires and obtain your scores for all specialties online at http://www.sdn.net, or compare your job values (as recorded in the Appendix) with the job values of urologists:

Urologists' Choices:	My Choices:
1. Variety	1. _____
2. Achievement	2. _____
2. Working with people	3. _____
2. Independence	4. _____

(there is a three-way tie for second place)

No one chose: Sufficient time off, feedback from others, prestige.

Summary Profile of Urologists   **My Personal Profile as an Urologist**
(derived from questionnaire answers)

They tend to:	I tend to: (circle one number)				
	Never	Rarely	Sometimes	Frequently	Always
Become bored with repetitive activity	1	2	3	4	5
Value independence highly	1	2	3	4	5
Enjoy being an "expert"	1	2	3	4	5
Have manual dexterity	1	2	3	4	5
Need to see tangible results of their efforts quickly	1	2	3	4	5
Prefer a planned schedule	1	2	3	4	5
Be energized by people	1	2	3	4	5
Be outgoing	1	2	3	4	5
Be uncomfortable with poorly defined problems	1	2	3	4	5
Be achievers	1	2	3	4	5

Add total of numbers circled to get your TOTAL SCORE: _____

Transfer score to the Appendix.

Urology

    sounds like me _____

    could be a possibility _____

    doesn't sound like me at all _____

PART 3

EMERGING
SPECIALTY AREAS

Subspecialties and EpiSpecialty Areas

ALL OF YOU WILL BEGIN YOUR RESIDENCY TRAINING IN ONE of the specialties recognized by the American Board of Medical Specialties and described in Part 2 of this book. However, after completing basic residency training, an increasing number of physicians are branching out in a variety of career directions—what I am calling epispecialties. This is a neologism describing special areas of expertise often with certificates of added qualifications or other formal attestations of expertise. This does not refer to those starting a second residency in another field, but rather those building on the skills and knowledge gained during residency years. Some are motivated by personal interests outside of medicine, such as performing arts or competitive sports; others, by populations served in their geographic location, such as the elderly in a retirement community or students in private school or college setting. Your original desire to be a physician may be related to an interest in women's health, addiction problems in society, or the medical needs of immigrants. During residency or practice years, you may discover that you have unexpected talent in a field such as administrative medicine.

There are opportunities to practice in specific settings—international medicine, as a full- or part-time medical missionary or a consultant to an international agency for health development; the travel industry, as the physician on adventure tours or cruise ships; a pharmaceutical company, as a clinical researcher; an institution, such as a prison; the media, as a journalist or radio/television consultant; or federal or state government, as a health policy analyst. All these opportunities are open to physicians from a variety of specialty backgrounds. Whatever you choose as a specialty generally does not limit you to one practice style or setting.

On the basis of students' suggestions, seven "emerging" epispecialty areas are discussed in Part 3: addiction, administrative, adolescent, critical care, geriatrics, hospice and palliative, and sports medicine. Many current residents and practicing physicians are incorporating these aspects of medicine into their practices. None is recognized as a separate specialty by the American Board of Medical Specialties (ABMS), which grants approval to a new board upon demonstration of a body of knowledge that can be taught, tested, and practiced. ABMS policy is, "They must demonstrate that it is a new field of medical science, and not just a new technique, that there are a sizable number of residency programs in that field, and that a sizable group of physicians limit their practice to that field." The creation of a new ABMS board also must be supported by specialty societies in the field.[1]

REFERENCE

1.   Pinkney DS. Specialty board in addiction medicine eyed. AMNews 1990;33:9-10.

Addiction Medicine

"We feel that addiction medicine has to be recognized at this time because the nation needs it. . . . Addiction affects, on a day-to-day basis, probably 30 to 50 percent of everything that a doctor sees."

—Jess Bromley, M.D.[2]

FAST FACTS:

Number of accredited fellowship programs in addiction psychiatry: 40

Number of positions available in 2009: 64

Length of training: 1-2 years (after 4 year psychiatry residency)

Competitiveness Ranking: Low

Number in US certified by the American Board of Psychiatry and Neurology in Addiction Psychiatry: approximately 1,200

Number in US certified by the American Society of Addiction Medicine in 2008: 4,200[1]

Mean of net income after expenses, before taxes: lower than $194,400 reported for all MDs

Mean number of hours weekly for patient care and professional activities: varies with practice setting

There are physicians who devote a large part or even all of their practices to treating patients with alcohol and drug addiction problems. More than 3500 physicians are members of the American Society of Addiction Medicine (ASAM). This organization has developed a certification procedure (not recognized by the American Board of Medical Specialties) based on a physician's professional experience with a written examination to document expertise in drug and alcohol dependence.

What Are the Pathways to a Career in Addiction Medicine?

Most of the applicants for ASAM certification are trained in family medicine, general internal medicine, psychiatry, pediatrics, and obstetrics and gynecology.[3]

To gain expertise in addiction medicine, physicians report they have taken educational courses and joined related professional societies. Although medical education lacks systematic training in addiction medicine, there are post-residency fellowship programs in addiction psychiatry. The American Board of Psychiatry and Neurology together with the American Psychiatric Association has developed a Certificate of Added Qualifications in Addiction Psychiatry that is approved by the American Board of Medical Specialties and requires an additional year of residency training. Also, both the Psychiatry and Internal Medicine Residency Review Committees have mandated training in alcoholism and addictions during residency. Currently, approximately 1200 certificates have been issued in addiction psychiatry.

Types of Practice. Most physicians practice addiction medicine as part of their regular medical practice, and they offer education on potential addiction dangers to all patients as well as treating alcoholism and other drug dependencies in those who are addicted. One physician sees his role as ". . . seeing patients who don't know they're alcoholic or don't know they have a problem yet. . . ."[4] You may become so well-known as an "expert" in this area that you find that other physicians refer substance abuse patients to you and your "nonaddictive" patients seek care elsewhere. Partners in your practice should share your interest; additional counselors or psychologists might be added as staff.

Some physicians direct drug and alcohol treatment center programs on a full- or part-time basis. These programs, set up on an inpatient or outpatient basis, often involve other health care professionals, such as psychologists, social workers, and occupational therapists. However, cost containment pressures have led to the closure of many inpatient programs, and managed care has forced innovation and efficiency.[5]

What Abilities and Talents are Important in Addiction Medicine?

"Persistence and the ability to work for a long time without any tangible results" is the most commonly stated answer. Also, training in behavioral and biomedical aspects of medicine is imperative. The physician needs to be able to build an atmosphere of trust with patients and their families. To work in a treatment center, you will need to develop administrative and teamwork skills, learn how to conduct a meeting, delegate tasks, write grants to secure funding, and organize daily activities efficiently.

What Personality Traits Best Characterize Addiction Medicine Physicians?

Respondents say they want to "understand" people and enjoy "becoming part of a patient's life," but, at the same time, "I need to stay objective and not become too involved." In addition, they are challenged by the multifaceted aspects of substance abuse: "It's like putting together pieces of a puzzle."

What Advice Would You Give a Medical Student Interested in Addiction Medicine?

"I would urge that you examine your reasons for your interest—you need to know that you are not going to have a lot of successes and won't be able to save everyone." Students are advised to take courses in counseling techniques, especially in the area of family therapy.

What Are the Future Challenges to Addiction Medicine?

"To get better training for all physicians in this area—not just those who have a special interest, but for everyone." "We need motivated teachers to overcome the natural reluctance of medical students to engage in activities that are beyond their control or without a quick solution."

"A major factor is that many physicians and nurses come from alcoholic homes . . . (they) don't recognize (it) as a problem because it was something they grew up with. They have their own blinders."[2] "Fear of losing patients is a major barrier to identifying an addiction problem. . . . If you get rejected by a patient, that hurts."[2]

Increasingly, primary care physicians are seeing individuals with substance use disorders, but there is little guidance on how to develop models of care and collaboration with others in the health care system.[6] In addition, there has been a decline in the number of psychiatrists training in addiction psychiatry.[7]

RESOURCES

The American Society of Addiction Medicine, 4601 North Park Avenue, Suite 101, Upper Arcade, Chevy Chase, MD 20815. Telephone: (301) 656-3920. Internet address: www.asam.org.

REFERENCES

1. ASAM News , April 2008, Vol 23, No 2. Accessed at www.asma. org January 10, 2011.
2. Bromley J, quoted in Pinkney DS. Specialty board in addiction medicine eyed. *Amer Med News* 1990;33(22):9–10.
3. Stevens S. Looking forward to the 21st Century. *Young Physicians* 1998;2(6):29.
4. Swander H. Addiction medicine is growing part of family practice. *AAFP Reporter* 1991;18(2):1,6.
5. Hearn W. Managed addiction. *Amer Med News* 1995;38:17–18, 23–24.

6. Stein MD, Friedmann PD. Generalist physicians and addiction care. *JAMA* 2001;286(14):1764-1765.

7. Soyka M, Gorelick DA. Why should addiction medicine be an attractice field for young physicians? *Addiction* 2009 Feb:104(2):169-172.

Administrative Medicine

BECOMING A "PHYSICIAN-EXECUTIVE"—MOVING FROM "THE bedside to the boardroom"—is the logical consequence of the "corporatization" of medicine. Dr. David Nash says that hospitals and managed care organizations are looking for physician-executives "who can speak the language of finance and management and the language of clinical care."[1]

In 1975, there were 64 members of the American Academy of Medical Executives. The American College of Physician Executives (ACPE) with over 9,000 members is a fast growing physician group. Since January 1997, the American Board of Medical Management has approved 1,486 Certified Physician Executives,[2] but this certification is not currently approved by the American Board of Medical Specialties.

What Are the Pathways to a Career in Administrative Medicine?

The number of joint MD/MBA programs at medical schools has increased from 28 in 1997 to 65 today.[3] Courses are taken in the summers before and after the first year of medical school and during the third and fourth years so that the dual-degree program does not prolong medical training.

Physicians are entering Master of Business Administration (MBA) programs and majoring in health care administration—a commitment of two to three years. Other options are to receive a Master of Medical Management (MMM) or a Master of Health Administration (MHA) degree. A mid-career physician can enroll in a more flexible medical administration graduate program at a university, attending classes part-time, on weekends, or via computer home-study. Courses are typical of business school – finance, accounting, management theory – but they emphasize how to use this information in health care settings.

All types of specialty physicians are pursuing this pathway, but it seems particularly appealing to those with a generalist frame of reference who are intrigued by the management and financial aspects of practice. In addition, it is helpful to have five to ten years of practice experience so that you know what you need to know.

Types of Practice. "This isn't a part-time job anymore . . . physicians aren't going in and working as administrators one day a week. Now they're a vital part of the management team."[4] You can be a physician manager in a group practice; a managed-care program, such as a health maintenance organization (HMO), preferred provider organization (PPO), or managed fee-for-service entity; academic medical center; or hospital. Third-party payers and large corporations are looking for physician-executives to manage medical care for groups of employees.

Some physicians wish to maintain their clinical practice—one respondent spends about 30 percent of his time as a group practice manager and the rest in family medicine, "I still enjoy being a doctor. I don't want to lose that."[4]

Although financial rewards are not the primary reason for the surge of interest in administrative medicine, most physician-executives are earning more than they could in full-time clinical practice. Average starting salary for the MD/MBA is $292,500, higher than the $192,196 average income for a medical specialist without an MBA.[3]

What Abilities and Talents Are Important in Administrative Medicine?

"You need to be able to see both the clinical and business side of running a practice." "If we're looking at mammography equipment,

I can look at it from a clinical perspective as well as from a capital investment perspective."[4]

Most mid-career physician-executives report that they "fell into administration by default—the business side was being ignored and no one else seemed to be able to handle it." An individual's organizational talent must be augmented with formal training in management, motivation, and negotiation skills. Presentation skills with proficiency in using spreadsheet software and making data "meaningful to colleagues" are essential.[5] In addition, you have to be able to delegate tasks comfortably because much of your interaction involves groups or teams.

What Personality Traits Best Characterize Administrative Medicine Physicians?

A nontraditional business personality seems to choose this career track—more of a "visionary" than a "manager." Physician-executives want to have more impact on society than is possible in one-to-one patient encounters. They describe themselves as future-oriented and able to see problems as multifaceted challenges: "I can look at any capital project from the angles of acquisition costs, depreciation, use-debt capacity, working capital, and so on. I can understand the health of the company and the prospects for its future."[4]

One respondent was attracted to administrative medicine in order to "gain some physician control over the increasingly bureaucratic world of medicine." This need for control is congruent with findings of Myers-Briggs studies on physicians who are attracted to administrative work settings. These individuals tend to live their lives in a structured, orderly manner and are uncomfortable with ambiguity.

However, another side emerges in administrative medicine: "It's a new need and necessary dimension to health care management. We need to have health care leaders firmly fixed on the patient and quality and not on the bottom line. Physicians understand health care needs better than other kinds of purely business-trained managers."[4]

What Advice Would You Give a Medical Student Interested in Administrative Medicine?

Few students or even residents initially intend to become physician-executives. Most see themselves as clinicians, not administrators. However, with increasing awareness of the future trends in medicine toward managed care and opportunities during training to spend time in ambulatory care settings away from the medical school, students see the need to learn more about the business side of medicine.

In addition to "challenging the medical curriculum to integrate exposure to "real-life" economic, business, and legal aspects of medicine," students are advised to become active in organizational activities within or outside the medical school. Such involvement will afford "on-the-job training" in negotiation, communication, and organizational skills. One physician became interested in administrative medicine after serving as president of his house-staff association in which he sat on the hospital's medical-policy committee. He observed "constant battles over resources and institutional policy, and it was frustrating to witness the lack of leadership on the part of the physicians."[6]

What Are the Future Challenges to Administrative Medicine?

If physicians are to have a say in the future direction of health care, more physicians must commit to a full-time career in administrative medicine. "What will be required is physicians in areas of management responsibility that go beyond quality assurance or medical staff affairs and that include having a real voice in resource allocation and the nature of contracts with third-party payers."[7]

Physicians must help develop information systems for quality assurance, benefit packages for sponsored care of patients, and health care systems to meet societal needs.

RESOURCES

The American College of Physician Executives, 400 North Ashley Drive, Suite 400, Tampa, FL 33602. Telephone: (800) 562-8088. Internet address: www.acpe.org.

National Association of MD/MBA Students, http://www.md-mba. org/ founded in 2004, has a listing of programs at http://www.md-mba. org/programs.html#us

REFERENCES

1. Nash DB, quoted in Thomas P. Demand for doctor managers booms in HMOs and hospitals. *Med World News,* June 12, 1989, p. 29.
2. www.ccmm.org, accessed January 21, 2011.
3. Butcher L. The rapid growth of MD/MBA programs: Are they worth it? PEJ Jan-Feb 2011:pp.22-26.
4. Archbold C. Growing number of physician executives assuming health care leadership roles. *Physician Finan News,* February 28, 1989, pp. 1, 36.
5. Cejka S. Don't buy these myths about a medical management job. *Med Economics* 1998;75(5):38–40.
6. Hodge RH Jr., Nash DB. The physician-executive. In: *Future practice alternatives in medicine,* Nash DB, ed. New York: Igaku-Shoin, 1987, pp. 236, 262.
7. Heyssel RM. Administrative medicine. *JAMA* 1990;263(19):2620.

Adolescent Medicine

FAST FACTS:

Number of accredited fellowship programs: 27

Number of fellows in training: 67

Competitiveness Ranking: Low

Length of training: 2-3 years (after three year residency in family medicine, internal medicine or pediatrics)

Number in US certified in specialty: 55 (family medicine), 38 (internal medicine), 547 (pediatrics)

Median compensation for all physicians in specialty: less than the $180,000 for pediatricians

Mean number of hours weekly for patient care and professional activities: lower than 54.1 reported for all MDs

INTEREST IN ADOLESCENT MEDICINE AS A SEPARATE SPECIALTY of medicine is not new. The first adolescent unit was established in 1952 by J. Roswell Gallagher, M.D., at Boston Children's Hospital with the rationale that "medical clinics devoted to the care of a single age group foster a physician's tendency to consider his patient, diminish the likelihood that he will focus upon disease alone, and help to increase his knowledge of what patients are like and what they require at various times of their lives."[1] Sixteen years later, the Society for Adolescent Medicine was established, and in 1972 the American Academy of Pediatrics issued a policy statement that claimed adolescents as part of the patient group served by pediatricians.[2]

What Are the Pathways to a Career in Adolescent Medicine?

Adolescent medicine has been approved as a subspecialty of family medicine, pediatrics, and internal medicine. The first certification examination was offered in 1994 and was administered conjointly by the American Board of Pediatrics and the American Board of Internal Medicine. The American Board of Family Medicine joined the other two boards in offering the same examination for the first time in November 2001. Board certified family physicians qualified either through completion of two years of fellowship training or a practice pathway were eligible to take the examination. The practice pathway expired after the 2005 examination.[3] There are 489 pediatricians, 55 family physicians, and 68 internists who have earned Certificates of Added Qualifications,[4] but not all certifications are still valid.

There are 27 accredited adolescent medicine fellowship programs, offering two-three years of training after completion of three years of family medicine, pediatrics, or internal medicine training. Of the 60 current fellows, 83.3% are women.[5] The Society for Adolescent Health and Medicine is a multispecialty organization committed to improving the physical and psychosocial health and well being of all adolescents.

Types of Practice. Few physicians in private practice focus exclusively on the care of adolescents. Most treat adolescents as part of their regular pediatric, internal medicine, or family medicine practice. However, a physician may become known as an "expert" in dealing with adolescents and treat a growing percentage of patients in this age range. Those in academics or salaried positions are more likely to financially be able to limit their clinical focus to adolescents. Sixty-five percent of recent fellowship graduates have become full-time faculty members.

A major disincentive to the full-time practice of adolescent medicine has been the low level of reimbursement for time spent with patients in counseling and education. In addition, many adolescents have not had health insurance.[6]

What Abilities and Talents Are Important in Adolescent Medicine?

In addition to the abilities and talents needed to practice pediatrics, family medicine, and general internal medicine, it is important to be comfortable with teenagers and to be patient: "You've got to take a flexible approach to their problems; you have to have the willingness to spend time with them."[7]

Respondents say that treating adolescents is often more difficult than treating adults: teenagers question therapy more, and negotiation may be necessary so parents feel comfortable about not being consulted about all aspects of their adolescent's care. Training in behavioral medicine and communication skills is especially important in this field.

Physicians need to feel comfortable working with nurse practitioners, physician assistants, counselors, and other health care providers to improve the health of adolescents.

What Personality Traits Best Characterize Adolescent Medicine Physicians?

All respondents indicate that even though it is important to be open to new ideas and flexible in dealing with adolescents, an organized and structured approach to problem solving is most helpful. One respondent says: "Offering logical choices to adolescents can be very helpful and nonthreatening."

Other traits include being "nonjudgmental," "empathetic," and "able to laugh at yourself." You also need to be able to look at the "big picture" because the adolescent's family and environment impact on health status. Dr. Carolyn Lopez, a family physician at a public hospital in Chicago, says, "be more of a listener than a talker."[8]

What Advice Would You Give a Medical Student Interested in Adolescent Medicine?

"Seek extra training in counseling and patient education techniques, since these areas are not emphasized in the traditional medical school curriculum and, even if you don't focus on adolescent medicine in the future, you'll find the skills helpful in dealing with people."

"Spend time with adolescents to be sure that your expectations are not unrealistic."

What Are the Future Challenges to Adolescent Medicine?

Respondents agree that it is necessary to counter the feeling of helplessness when dealing with adolescents. Solutions will not come overnight, and Americans are uncomfortable without immediate solutions to problems associated with teenage pregnancy, drug abuse, alcoholism, suicide, tobacco use, and accidents.

The danger in designating adolescent medicine as a separate subspecialty is that it will not be seen as the responsibility of all physicians, but rather the "problem" to be solved by the "experts." Strasburger says, "What would be gratifying would be for the medical profession . . . to embrace wholeheartedly the idea of adolescent medicine . . . so that more about adolescence is taught and *all* physicians learn how to care for and cope with teenagers."[1]

Another respondent says, "In the current system of managed care, there are many barriers to improving adolescent care. We are pressured to see more patients, have shorter visits, and are not well reimbursed for prevention efforts. However, managed care may ultimately be the driving force in requiring health screening for pregnancy prevention, substance use, and mental health issues."

RESOURCE

The Society for Adolescent Health and Medicine, 111 Deer Lake Road, Ste 100, Deerfield, Illinois 60015. Telephone: (847)753-5226. Internet address: www.adolescenthealth.org.

REFERENCES

1. Strasburger VC. Who speaks for the adolescent? *JAMA* 1983;249(8):1021.

2. American Academy of Pediatrics: Policy statement. *Pediatrics* 1972;49:463.

3. Certificate of Added Qualifications in Adolescent Medicine. *JABFP* 2001;14(2):159-161.

4. https://www.abp.org/abpwebsite/stats/wrkfrc/workforce09.pdf, accessed January 21, 2011.

5. Graduate Medical Education, 2009-2010. *JAMA* 2009;304(11):1257.

6. Blum RW. Society for Adolescent Medicine inaugural speech. *J Adol Med* 1991;12:408–411.

7. Glasbrenner K. Physicians taking adolescent medicine from benches to trenches. *JAMA* 1986;255(4):441–443.

8. Quoted in Gabriel J. For teens, the issue is trust. *Parade Magazine*, September 15, 2002, p. 7.

Critical Care Medicine

FAST FACTS:

Number of fellowship positions to be offered in 2009: 221

Competitiveness Ranking: Very high

Length of training: 1-3 years after residency

Number of fellowship programs: 45 (anesthesiology), 32 (internal medicine), 61 (pediatrics), 94 (surgery), 152 (pulmonary), 25 (neuro)

Number of fellows in training: 62 (anesthesiology), 136 (internal medicine), 357 (pediatrics), 152 (surgery), 1,266 (pulmonary)

Number in US certified in specialty: 953 (anesthesiology), 7,791 (internal medicine), 991 (pediatrics), 1,835 (surgery)

Median compensation for all physicians in specialty: $215,462

Mean number of hours weekly for patient care and professional activities: higher than 51.6 reported for all MDs

"A MULTIDISCIPLINARY ENDEAVOR THAT CROSSES TRADITIONAL departmental and specialty lines" and ". . . a discipline, based in the intensive care unit of a hospital, with its primary concern being the care of the patient with a critical illness" are two descriptions of critical care medicine.[1] In its broadest sense, critical care medicine includes transportation to the hospital, time in the emergency room, the operating room and, eventually, the intensive care or coronary care unit.[2]

Initially, the care of critically ill and injured patients evolved in an unstructured manner, with hospitals training personnel as new technology was developed.

What Are the Pathways to a Career in Critical Care Medicine?

In the early 1980s, there was an effort to conjointly offer certification in critical care for physicians from many specialties, but a common examination could not be written. In 1986, the American Board of Medical Specialties approved a certification of special competence in critical care for the boards in internal medicine, anesthesiology, pediatrics and surgery.[3] Fellowship training from six months to three years in length is available to physicians who have completed a primary residency training, such as three years of internal medicine or five years of general surgery. Most critical care physicians are internists, usually pulmonologists who may incorporate their critical care training into their three-year pulmonary diseases fellowship, leading to dual subspecialty certification. Surgeons may obtain training in critical care combined with trauma or burn care. A few anesthesiology residency programs are integrating primary training in anesthesiology with advanced critical care training in a four to five-year program, eliminating the need to go through a fellowship program.[4]

The American College of Emergency Physicians' Critical Care Committee issued a position paper "The Future of Critical Care Medicine Within Emergency Medicine" that urged subspecialty postgraduate training in critical care medicine for emergency physicians. This training would emphasize prehospital and emergency department care rather than preparation for care of hospitalized patients.[5] The American Board of Emergency Medicine (ABEM) and the American Board of Internal Medicine (ABIM) have joined together to offer a five-year combined program with three years of primary emergency medicine followed by two years of medicine critical care with certification by the ABIM.[4]

Types of Practice. Many critical care physicians continue to practice in their primary specialty while also caring for their hospital intensive care unit patients. Large hospitals may have separate divisions of critical care medicine that employ physicians with expertise in this field on a full-time basis.

What Abilities and Talents Are Important in Critical Care Medicine?

Critical care is a "multisystem field"—internists need experience in postoperative care and trauma, anesthesiologists need medical and cardiac intensive care training. One respondent says, "the problems of critically ill patients are not specialty-based: chronic disease aspects appeal to the internists; reflex activity appeals to the anesthesiologists. You need to have the ability to sit and reflect plus the technical expertise to take action." Another says, "It helps to like procedures and have good manual skills."

What Personality Traits Best Characterize Critical Care Physicians?

One respondent calls his colleagues "showmen" who are aggressive people. He describes himself as "liking catastrophes." Decisiveness is cited as an important trait. Because of the need to work as a team with other health professionals in the intensive care unit, often seeking consultation from other subspecialists, it is "important to get along with people."

What Are the Future Challenges to Critical Care Medicine?

The debate over certification among a variety of specialties led to the agreement that formalized training is needed for this area of medicine—all subspecialists in this field need additional training in special skills and knowledge, and curriculums need to be developed.

One respondent says, "The academic growth of critical care medicine will proceed slowly until those formally trained become leaders in departments sponsoring certification. If critical care physicians see themselves as primarily pulmonologists or anesthesiologists—with extra training in critical care medicine—full specialty status will never be attained for critical care medicine."

"Ideally, there would be interdepartmental cooperation in training programs rather than various specialties offering parallel programs leading to certification."

Another challenge is whether critical care will appeal to physicians as they age. Respondents say that this is a high stress, high burnout field that requires youthful energy and endurance. Like emergency medicine, this field lacks role models who have practiced critical care as a full-time career for more than 15 to 20 years.

RESOURCES

American Society of Critical Care Anesthesiologists, 520 N. Northwest Highway, Park Ridge, Illinois 60068. Telephone: 847-825-5586. Internet address: www.ascca.org

The Society of Critical Care Medicine, 500 Midway Drive, Mount Prospect, Illinois 60056. Telephone: (847) 827-6869. Internet address: www.sccm.org. Student membership is available.

REFERENCES

1. Shapiro BA. Critical care medicine. *JAMA* 1982;247(21):2945.
2. What makes a critical care unit? *Emer Med* September 30, 1983, p. 166.
3. Kelley MA. Sounding board. Critical care medicine—a new specialty? *N Engl J Med* 1988;318(24):1613–1616.
4. Hartsell T. Fellow program directors' breakfast. ASCCA Interchange, Anes & Analgesia, 2010; 21(1):7.
5. Falk JL. The future of critical care medicine within emergency medicine. *Ann Emer Med* 1991;20(3):320–321.

Geriatrics

IN RESPONSE TO THE RAPIDLY AGING POPULATION, THE FIELD of geriatrics has emerged as a special area of expertise. While most care of the elderly will continue to be provided by primary care physicians—the family physician and general internist—all physicians will treat an increased number of elderly patients. One estimate is that by the year 2030, one in five Americans (20 percent) will be over the age of 65.[1]

What Are the Pathways to a Career in Geriatric Medicine?

In 1978, the Institute of Medicine of the National Academy of Science recommended that a "formal practice specialty in geriatrics not be established, but that gerontology and geriatrics be recognized as academic disciplines within relevant medical specialties."[2] In 1988, the American Boards of Internal Medicine and Family Practice jointly sponsored an examination for those certified in either specialty leading to the granting of a Certificate of Added Qualifications in Geriatric Medicine; the certificate is valid for a 10-year period. The purpose of certification, according to Benson,[3] is not to identify and isolate doctors competent to treat the elderly, but rather to stimulate teaching and research and to reward physicians who have developed geriatric expertise in their own clinical practices. Murray adds that "one of the positive things to emerge from the certification process was that it spurred physicians to take courses in geriatrics."[4]

The practice pathway to certification ended in 1994. Now, you have to complete a one-year geriatric medicine fellowship to qualify for certification. Many programs have an additional one- to two-year track for those interested in academics or research. In addition, there are two-year fellowships in geriatric psychiatry.

Types of Practice. Some feel that board-certified geriatricians should focus on research, medical education, consultation, and administration. Others call for intensified efforts to increase the numbers of clinical geriatricians to meet the projected needs of primary health care to the elderly.[5] Full-time geriatric practice opportunities will be developed as geriatric outpatient and assessment clinics are established in urban centers. In certain geographic locations, such as Florida or Arizona, there will be a disproportionate number of elderly patients and this may attract clinical geriatricians. Opportunities for geriatricians are plentiful in managed care. Special programs such as the Program of All-Inclusive Care of the Elderly (PACE) recruit geriatricians. Many staff-model Health Maintenance Organizations or large group practices hire geriatricians to manage the frail elders and those in nursing homes and subacute care units.

However, the vast majority of family physicians and general internists will continue to grow old with their patients, offering continuous comprehensive care. Some may incorporate patient care in a nursing home or retirement center into their existing practices. Most people believe it is unrealistic to expect there will be enough trained geriatricians in the United States to take care of all elderly patients: "You're simply not going to take care of 25 million elderly people with a few thousand certified geriatricians."[5]

Reimbursement for geriatric care is relatively low, with patients requiring time, both in examination procedures and in communication. In addition, those who treat the elderly often grapple with the bureaucracy of Medicare's billing system. The Resource-Based Relative Value Scale (RBRVS) is looked to as a hope for improved compensation for primary care physicians providing geriatric care. On the other hand, in managed care, geriatrics can be used to reduce high costs of care for the frail elders, a group well known for high rates of utilization. Rather than expecting them to "pay their way" with fee-for-service billings, geriatricians can be financed by the savings their care creates.

What Abilities and Talents Are Important in Geriatric Medicine?

"There are definite skills that are unique to dealing with the elderly—history taking is more complicated in terms of the patient's memory and past reactions to illness; physical examination requires specific techniques not necessary in the younger patient; and communication may be complicated by hearing or visual loss."

Some feel it is easier to understand the elderly if you are elderly yourself: "I have been in practice for 40 years and my patients are my contemporaries and my friends—they came to me when they and I were young. Now I guess you'd say I have a geriatric practice."

"You have to accept your own aging process." A number of younger respondents admitted that it was hard not to be influenced by societal negativity about aging and the futility of treating disease in an elderly person.

"An enthusiasm for dealing with families is crucial. Families provide 85 percent of the care to frail elderly and the physician is their main resource."

What Personality Traits Best Characterize Geriatricians?

"You need to be content with small successes—not dramatic results." Geriatricians are also described as "team players," able to work closely with nurses, therapists, nutritionists, and social workers. "Those who have a need to understand and comfort people will find satisfaction in geriatrics." "It's important to treat the 'whole person,' not just focus on the disease."

What Advice Would You Give a Medical Student Interested in Geriatric Medicine?

Many respondents described geriatric medicine as a new "frontier." One advised, "Think of the future opportunities when it is estimated that 75 percent of almost every physician's practice will involve contact with patients over the age of 65—and you have the training and credentials in geriatrics." Learn as much as you can about normal aging, diseases that affect the elderly, and pharmacology for this age group."

Ethical issues are also important. In geriatrics, the problem is not what the physician *can* do but what the physician *should* do. Doctors must learn to be proactive in discussing treatment preference in advance. Sensitivity and compassion are critical attributes of the physician caring for older people.

What Are the Future Challenges to Geriatric Medicine?

There seems to a need for more physicians interested in geriatrics, particularly to become academicians and serve as role models for students. To address this, the first Combined Internal Medicine-Geriatric Medicine residency program started in July 2002 at the Medical College of Wisconsin, offering a longitudinal experience in geriatrics for four years.

Within the field itself, there are active areas of research in basic sciences, particularly in the primary dementias; problems of the frail elderly and prevention strategies; and health services in a time of cost containment.[6]

"Perhaps the greatest challenge will be balancing the needs of individual patients with the need to control the rise of health care spending. The burden of illness is high in a portion of the elderly population. Almost 60 percent of all Medicare dollars are spent on approximately 10 percent of the older population. Physicians, patients, families, and communities need to develop ways to ensure high quality care at a reasonable cost to our society."

RESOURCE

The American Geriatrics Society, 350 Fifth Ave., Suite 801, New York, NY 10001. Telephone: (212) 308-1414. Internet address: www. americangeriatrics.org. Free student membership is available. There is a trainee link with information on mentoring programs and the student and resident chapter network.

REFERENCES

1. *Vision for the future*. New York: American Geriatrics Society, 1998.
2. Schneider EL, Butler RN. Geriatrics. *JAMA* 1981;245(21):2190–2191.
3. Benson JA. Quoted in Taylor M. What does the geriatrics exam mean to you? *Senior Patient,* September/October 1989, pp. 65–67.
4. Murray J. Quoted in Cogen J. Certificates for FPs gain momentum. *Fam Prac News* 1988;18(14):41.
5. List ND. We need more geriatricians. Letters. *JAMA* 1994;272(11):847.
6. Applegate WB, Pahor M. Geriatric medicine. *JAMA* 1997;277(23):1863–1864.

Hospice and Palliative Care

FAST FACTS:

Number of fellowship programs accredited by ACGME: 73

Number of fellowship programs accredited by AOA: 3

Competitiveness Ranking: Low

Length of training: 1 year after residency

Number certified by the American Board of Hospice and Palliative Care from 1996 to 2006: 2,883

Number certified by the American Board of Medical Specialties from 2008-2010: 1,271

Mean of net income: lower than $194,400 reported for all MDs

Mean number of hours weekly for patient care and professional activities: higher than 51.6 reported for all MDs

USED AS EARLY AS THE 1500S, THE WORD "PALLIATE" MEANS "treatment when cure is not possible." Derived from the Latin *pallium,* meaning a "mantle, cloak, or cover," and the late Latin *palliatus,* "to relieve without curing,"[1] hospice and palliative medicine has become a valid and essential component of today's care of the dying patient. A recognized medical specialty in the United Kingdom, Australia, and New Zealand, palliative care has been endorsed by the Institute of Medicine report, *Approaching Death: Improving Care at the End of*

Life,[2] as a discipline that "should become, if not a medical specialty, at least a defined area of expertise, education and research."

Under the World Health Organization (WHO) Expert Committee's definition, palliative medicine is limited to noncurative care of the dying patient. The emphasis shifts from prolonging life to relieving suffering and controlling symptoms. Management plans need to be individualized according to the patient's wishes. The focus is on comprehensive care, including cultural, social, psychological, ethical, and spiritual aspects. Interdisciplinary teamwork is a key feature of palliative medicine, with the physician's role as one member of the team.[3]

What Are the Pathways to a Career in Hospice and Palliative Medicine?

One-year of fellowship training is available and, after 2012, will be mandatory for certification in this field. There are 10 co-sponsoring American Board of Medical Specialties (ABMS) boards and 3 American Osteopathic Association (AOA) boards. Internal medicine and family medicine are the most common pathways, but fellowships are available for those who are ABMS board-certified or board eligible in anesthesiology, emergency medicine, pediatrics, physical medicine and rehabilitation, psychiatry and neurology, obstetrics-gynecology, radiology, and surgery; and AOA board-certified or board-eligible in family medicine, internal medicine, physical medicine and rehabilitation, and psychiatry and neurology.

Some advocate that all physicians should be trained to practice palliative medicine.[1] "In some sense it is nothing more than good basic medicine. I know lots of doctors—general internists, surgeons, oncologists—who do wonderful palliative care."[4] There are others who feel it should be a separate specialty with clear credentials and training programs.

Types of Practice. Most full-time palliative medicine physicians are employed by a hospice or academic center. One palliative care physician is a member of a multidisciplinary pain practice affiliated with an anesthesiology practice. Another is a partner in a medical oncology group practice.

What Abilities and Talents Are Important in Hospice and Palliative Medicine?

"The ability to relieve suffering" is the primary ability needed. In addition to physical pain, suffering refers to fear, anxiety, helplessness, hopelessness, humiliation, and various aspects of physical discomfort.[4] Much of the day is spent working with other health professionals in caring for patients and counseling family members; good team skills are needed. An awareness of and respect for cultural diversity and spirituality is imperative. Finally, a palliative medicine physician needs to develop an awareness of his or her own feelings about death and dying.

What Personality Traits Best Characterize Hospice and Palliative Medicine Physicians?

"Counselor types" are predominant in this field. Physicians who are able to give up control and allow the patient and family members to express their views are compatible with palliative medicine.

What Advice Would You Give a Medical Student Interested in Hospice and Palliative Care?

Interest in palliative care may be related to a medical student's own experience with the loss of a family member or friend. "It is important to get as much objective experience as possible, such as volunteering in a hospice program, to see how committed you are to the field." Students are also advised to get training in counseling techniques and ethical problem solving.

What Are the Future Challenges to Hospice and Palliative Medicine?

"Acceptance" by traditional medicine as a separate area of medicine is a challenge. Increased attention to hospice and palliative medicine in the United States is attributed to the "high cost of dying,"[5] attention to the role of medicine in caring rather than curing,[6] and the national debate on physician aid in dying. The issues related to economics and social policy will be a continuing challenge to physicians in this field.

Because the majority of people still die in hospitals, allowing payment for end-of-life care in this setting is an important challenge. However, creating a payment mechanism alone will not ensure that hospital-based palliative care would be provided in an appropriate nonmedical hospice model.[9]

RESOURCE

American Academy of Hospice and Palliative Medicine, 4700 W. Lake Ave., Glenview, IL 60025. Telephone: (847) 375-4712. Internet address: www.aahpm.org.

REFERENCES

1. Goodlin SJ. What is palliative care? *Hosp Pract* 1997;32(2):13.
2. Field MJ, Cassell CK. *Approaching death: Improving care at the end of life.* Institute of Medicine Committee on Care at the End of Life. Washington, DC: National Academy Press, 1997.
3. Fox E. Predominance of the curative model of medical care. Editorial. *JAMA* 1997;278(9):761–763.
4. Stollerman G. Palliative care and the suffering index. *Hosp Pract* 1997;32(2):19–21.
5. Scitovsky AA. The "high cost of dying" revisited. *Milbank Q* 1994;72:561–591.
6. Cassell EJ. The nature of suffering and the goals of medicine. *N Engl J Med* 1982;306:639–645.
7. Mahoney JJ. Correspondence. *N Engl J Med* 1997;336(14):1029.

Sports Medicine

MANY PHYSICIANS HAVE LABELED THEMSELVES "SPORTS medicine specialists" as Americans have become advocates of physical fitness. There is a need for physician involvement in fitness training, injury prevention, rehabilitation, and care of trauma. Bachman identifies all of the following specialists as having roles in sports medicine: "the family physician who knows the athlete's medical history and family makeup; the ophthalmologist who offers advice for eye protection and treatment; the internist for involved cardiac, metabolic, renal, or other problems; the dentist for mouth protection; the dermatologist for skin problems; the orthopaedist for musculoskeletal injuries; the psychologist or psychiatrist for psychological problems that frequently occur in athletes; the physical therapist and trainer, who are essential for prophylactic and therapeutic advice; the podiatrist for orthotics."[1] Primary care physicians and orthopaedists work together as team physicians on virtually all professional and college teams.[2] Sports medicine specialists deal with non-operative medical treatment of athletes while orthopaedic surgeons are also trained in the operative treatment of athletes' injuries. Approximately 90% of all sports injuries are non-surgical.[3]

You apply for a sports medicine fellowship at the beginning of your third year of residency, interview from September through December, and the match occurs in early January.

What Are the Pathways to a Career in Sports Medicine?

The widely varying certification programs offered by various sports organizations have led multidisciplinary groups to work together to develop standards in sports medicine for primary care physicians. The American Boards of Emergency Medicine, Family Medicine, Internal Medicine, Pediatrics, and Physical Medicine and Rehabilitation have offered conjointly a Certificate of Added Qualifications in Sports Medicine since 1993. Eighty percent of the almost 1300 certified physicians are family physicians.[4] It is necessary to complete a minimum of one year in an accredited sports medicine fellowship to qualify for certification. Currently, there are approximately 200 highly competitive fellowship programs.

Education, rather than certification, is the goal of the American Medical Society for Sports Medicine (AMSSM), an organization of nonsurgical physicians interested in sports medicine.

A listing of all fellowship programs and information on the application process is available from the website of the AMSSM.

Types of Practice. Most physicians interested in sports medicine incorporate it into their regular practices—serving as a volunteer team physician for the local high school, offering fitness evaluations and "exercise prescriptions" to patients seeking guidance, and treating recreational and competitive athletes for musculoskeletal injuries. An advocate of practicing sports medicine part-time says, "Don't turn your back on your discipline . . . to do sports medicine 100 percent of the time will cause you to lose your perspective."[2]

Financial rewards are not as great as people might think. Time spent in educating and counseling, especially if you are a team physician, does not receive appropriate compensation. Having a physical therapist on staff, however, can generate revenue. Physicians cite other rewards—the high motivation and appreciation of athlete-patients and involvement in something you understand and enjoy.

What Abilities and Talents Are Important in Sports Medicine?

Interest in sports medicine often arises from personal involvement in an individual or team sport. One respondent says, "Because I experience similar conditioning needs and often suffer comparable injuries, I'm more able to understand and work with a patient with a sports-related problem." Although personal sports activity is not essential, it does seem to enhance empathy for athletes. What are needed are counseling skills and an understanding of athletes' frustration when their activity is curtailed.

What Personality Traits Best Characterize Sports Medicine Physicians?

Respondents characterize themselves as "willing to take charge"; "able to see the big picture, rather than just the presenting symptoms;" and "motivators." "It is not enough to just tell the runner not to run— you need to be personally involved in helping your patient to adjust to the physical limitation." Another respondent says, "You need to have the patience to let time assist in healing many problems in sports medicine."

What Advice Would You Give a Medical Student Interested in Sports Medicine?

In addition to a good foundation in orthopaedics, you need to be a generalist. Training in cardiac testing, dermatology, nutrition, asthma management, and substance abuse counseling are recommended. It would be helpful to work with a local high school or college team physician, volunteering to assist with coverage of local athletic events or pre-participation sports examinations.

What Are the Future Challenges to Sports Medicine?

In the spring of 2011, sports medicine overcame one of its challenges. Medicare approved a specialty code for this specialty. This will allow physicians to negotiate with private payers on a variety of issues, ranging from reimbursement to privileges.[5] Quality assurance is being addressed by the formation of fellowship programs with the goal of academic legitimacy and research in the field.

The 2010 Socioeconomic and Health Policy Survey of the American Orthopaedic Society for Sports Medicine results[6] report an increase in treatment of individuals with osteoarthritis, both older and younger, and respondents anticipate increases in the use of viscosupplementation and decreases in bracing for treatment. Expected innovations in the near future are cartilage regeneration/repair as well as the development of biologics.

RESOURCES

The American College of Sports Medicine, 401 W. Michigan St., Indianapolis, IN 46202. Telephone: (317) 637-9200. Internet address: www.acsm.org.

The American Medical Society of Sports Medicine, 4000 West 114th Street, Suite 100, Leawood, Kansas 66211. Telephone: 913-327-1415. Internet address: www.amssm.org

The American Orthopaedic Society for Sports Medicine, 6300 N. River Road, Suite 500, Rosemont, Illinois 60018. Telephone: 847-292-4900. Internet; www.sportsmed.org

REFERENCES

1. Bachman WH. What is a sports medicine specialist? *AAFP Reporter* 1987;14(2):14.
2. Jancin B. FPs helped turn sports medicine into primary-care success story. *Fam Pract News* 1991;21(18):1, 52–53.
3. American Medical Society for Sports Medicine brochure, 2002.
4. Guardino J. Sports medicine a "blast," but not money driven. *Fam Pract News* 1998;28(5):80.
5. Madden C. Sports medicine assigned Medicare specialty code. The Sideline Report, August 2010, p.1.
6. Socioeconomic and Health Policy Survey Results, The American Orthopaedic Society for Sports Medicine, January 2010, p.24.

PART 4

PRACTICE OPTIONS

Practice Settings and Pathways

AS WE DISCUSS THEIR SPECIALTY INTERESTS, I ALSO ALWAYS ask students to think about where they want to live and how they want to use their medical degrees. Some of you have known since before admission to medical school exactly what you wish to do in medicine, not only in terms of your specialty, but also in terms of your practice setting. You may be planning to practice with a parent or local physician in your hometown after you finish residency. Perhaps you have already earned another degree, such as a PhD or JD, and your medical degree will enhance your abilities to secure an academic research position or to focus your legal practice on medical issues. More often, you may have a clear image of where you wish to live, for example, urban versus rural, but are not at all sure of what medical specialty would be the best for you. You may be sure that you will have a clinical practice but have not considered whether you would prefer the relative security of a negotiated salary and stated expectations or more financial risk and independence. Even in a clinical practice, you may be undecided as to whether you will be a hospital- or office-based physician.

Perhaps you would like to develop a personal interest, such as music, politics, or writing, as well as your career in medicine. Or you may be wondering if patient care is really what you want to do. A medical degree actually opens doors to a variety of opportunities. You could certainly choose to practice part-time while contributing to another field. Historically, there are many examples of such decisions. Oliver Wendell Holmes, Sr. had a faculty appointment at Harvard in the 1800s while pursuing his career as poet and philosopher. Nicolaus Copernicus, the 16th century astronomer, also served as physician to the Heilsberg Bishopric. Others completed medical school but eventually left medical practice for different careers, for example, in politics: Jean-Paul Marat of the French Revolution, Sun Yat-sen, the first president of the Chinese Republic, and Ernesto Che Guevara of Cuba; and in writing: Arthur Conan Doyle, Anton Chekhov, and A.J. Cronin. Another group also finished medical school but never practiced medicine: John Locke, the philosopher; Thomas Huxley, the biologist; and John Keats, W. Somerset Maugham, and Michael Crichton, writers.[1]

Currently, it is estimated that at least 20 percent of physicians are not involved in patient care; this number is expected to increase[2] and is certainly contributing to the increasing shortage of physicians. According to data from the 2010 AAMC Graduation Questionnaire, 31.1 percent of graduates plan to engage in full-time clinical practice, a decrease from 64.6 percent in 1990. In addition, a significant number of practicing physicians are taking "time off" or working part-time while pursuing personal interests.

In this section of the book I suggest possible career pathways, both clinical and non-clinical, and discuss how they relate to selecting a specialty. I also discuss how choosing among these many options will influence the geographic location in which you will live and work.

CLINICAL PATHWAYS

You definitely have decided that you will have a clinical practice. Today's clinical practice careers look very different from those of the past. Although private practice still continues to be the principal type of practice in the United States, managed care accelerated the move toward integrated group and salaried practice. However, more than a quarter of physicians still are self-employed in solo practice according to American Medical Association (AMA) data. Which financial form of practice to choose is an important determination, but more relevant to your specialty-choice decision is the setting in which you wish to practice. This is the decision that will be of major importance. Table 1 shows the specialties as they are most often practiced in an office- or hospital-based setting.

Table 1: Office-Based and Hospital-Based Practice Continuum

Office-Based Groups A	B	C	Hospital-Based D
Dermatology	Allergy & Immunology	Colon & Rectal Surgery	Anesthesiology
Medical Genetics	Cardiology	General Surgery	Emergency Medicine
Preventive Medicine	Endocrinology	Hematology	Nuclear Medicine
Rheumatology	Family Medicine	Infectious Diseases	Pathology
	Gastroenterology	Medical Oncology	Physical Medicine & Rehabilitation
	General Internal Medicine	Neurological Surgery	Radiation Oncology
	Nephrology	Obstetrics & Gynecology	Radiology, Diagnostic
	Neurology	Ophthalmology	
	Pediatrics, General	Orthopaedic Surgery	
	Psychiatry	Otolaryngology	
	Pulmonary Medicine	Pediatric Subspecialties	
		Plastic Surgery	
		Thoracic Surgery	
		Urology	

Office-Based Practice

You can practice full-time, part-time, or none of the time in an office-based (also called ambulatory care) setting, based upon your choice of specialty. The most recent AMA data show that of 740,867 physicians engaged in patient care, 556,818 are in office-based practices. Office-based settings include solo practice, group practice, and a staff-model Health Maintenance Organization (HMO). There are books and numerous articles in the literature about the relative benefits and disadvantages of the different models of private and salaried practice. However, regardless of the model of office-based practice you choose, your specialty choice will determine how much or how little time you will spend in this setting.

Almost all of the specialties in medicine can have an office component, especially as technology that was formerly used exclusively in hospitals becomes incorporated into office-based practices. An example of this is the prediction that in-office ultrasound will soon be affordable and part of the generalist's office practice. Physicians also will be doing much more disease-prevention and health-promotion work, an office-based activity.

Hospital-Based Practice

Traditional Hospital-Based Practice. Some physicians, such as surgeons, spend part of their time in the hospital and part in their private offices, providing pre- and post-operative care. However, in some specialties, you can be employed in a full-time hospital-based practice, receiving a salary from the hospital. You will be provided with an office and equipment, as well as some support staff. Hours may be more regular than if you were in an office-based practice, especially if you are in a non-direct patient care specialty, such as pathology or radiology. According to the AMA data, 75,976 U.S. physicians currently have a full time hospital-based practice.

Hospitalist. A new twist to choosing a specialty is the creation of the inpatient specialist or "hospitalist." This is considered to be the fastest growing specialty group in medicine with a current estimate of 20,000 physicians engaged in this work full-time. When the concept was introduced in 1996, most of the fewer than 1,000 hospitalists were trained in internal medicine; but now, pediatrician and family physicians have joined their ranks. Even obstetricians have a variation of this specialty with the introduction of "laborists," physicians whose sole role is to deliver babies in the hospital. It is estimated that approximately 85 percent of current hospitalists are trained in internal medicine.[3]

The particulars of the hospitalist system—the length of time on an inpatient service rotation, the interactions with the primary care physicians—vary from site to site. Hospitalists work in acute care medical wards, in intensive care units, and as medical consultants on surgical patients. One requirement is that there needs to be enough hospitalized patients to justify either a private group's or a hospital's hiring of a full-time hospitalist. More than one hospitalist also is needed to avoid individual burnout. Median salaries are reported to range from $160,000 for pediatricians to $218,000 for family physicians with employers subsidizing part since income from the care of an average of 12-15 patients daily cannot match this compensation.[4]

Some believe that the hospitalist role is an outgrowth of the emphasis of managed care on efficiency.[5] As long as generalists are caring for patients in both the office and hospital, there will be inherent time and effort conflicts. How to maintain the necessary skills for and be available to hospitalized patients is an increasing dilemma for physicians who spend most of their time in an office-based practice.

One physician who chose to leave office-based practice to become a hospitalist believes that it allows physicians to "employ integrated thinking by taking care of complex patients, experience a sense of closure on illness, and on a personal level, find a more defined role in terms of hours and physical setting."[6] He predicted that hospitalists will make up 20 percent of the internal medicine workforce in the 21st century and that there will be an "added qualifications" certification similar to those in geriatrics and sports medicine. This became reality in September 2009 when the American Board of Medical Specialties approved a "pilot program" for Recognition of Focused Practice (RFP) in Hospital Medicine. The American Boards of Internal Medicine and

Family Medicine have collaborated to offer certifying examinations; pediatrics might consider doing the same. The criteria are initial board certification in your respective specialty and practice experience focused on hospital medicine.[7] Information is available at the website for the Society of Hospital Medicine, www.hospitalmedicine.org.

Selected Patient Care Populations

Home Care. Once a major component of health care delivery, accounting for nearly half of all doctor-patient contact,[8] the house call was assumed to have disappeared. Although this is partially a myth because physicians do still go to patients' homes on occasion, the frequency has dramatically decreased over the past three decades.

There is now a resurgence of interest in home care, especially with the vast numbers of elderly in the current and future population. Call Doctor Medical Group of San Diego began 14 years ago to bring emergency room equipment to the home. Primary care is the service most offered by this group now, and physicians with broad-based clinical skills are most desired.[9] The American Academy of Home Care Physicians (www.aahcp.org) was successful in 1998 in convincing Medicare that an increase in reimbursement for house calls was justified, and payments were raised by as much as 50%.[8] An evolving innovation will be the "video house call," employing two-way video communications systems to maintain elderly patients in their homes rather than in nursing homes.

Performing Arts Medicine. Physicians who care for performers—dancers, singers, musicians—often share those interests themselves and need to have an understanding of the medical conditions and psychological stresses experienced by their patients. Physicians with a variety of specialty training backgrounds, including family medicine, internal medicine, neurology, physiatry, orthopaedic surgery, and rheumatology can care for this population, says one physician.[10] A few laryngologists have become noted for caring for vocalists. It is particularly important for the physician to be alert to the emotional reaction to the medical problem. "For symphony musicians, even the threat of a sore throat, nagging cough, or plugged ear is enough to send anxiety levels soaring," said the tour physician for the National Symphony Orchestra. He tallied 125 "office calls" in backstage corridors, hotel rooms, and airplanes.[11]

There currently are no fellowships in the field, and interested students are advised to spend some time with an experienced performing arts physician. There are a small number of performing arts clinics around the country, mostly in major cities with resident orchestras or ballet companies. There is a Performing Arts Medical Association, which offers student membership and publishes the journal, *Medical Problems of Performing Arts*.

Institutional Patient Care Positions

Academic Medicine. All specialties are found in academic medicine, and AMA data report 31,000 physicians in this setting. However, the emphasis is shifting from research and teaching to clinical care, and about half of the "Medical School" category physicians in the AMA data report that they are "office based." There is a need for primary care physicians in academic medicine to balance the subspecialists who have dominated the system. The development of non-tenured positions is a result of the pressure by managed care to generate patient care referrals to subspecialty colleagues and the need for revenue to support existing academic programs losing research funding.[12]

Federal Government. The U.S. Public Health Service (USPHS) Commissioned Corps, an all-officer uniformed service, and the Veterans Administration, serving war veterans both in ambulatory and hospital settings, employ many clinical physicians. The National Health Service Corps places physicians in underserved sites that are designated Health Manpower shortage areas. Within the USPHS, over 1000 physicians are engaged in patient care in the Indian Health Service (IHS). The internet address for the IHS is www.ihs.gov. Specifically, family physicians, internists, and psychiatrists are needed for underserved sites.

Military Medicine. In Part 5, there is a chapter on matching in a military residency program. A number of physicians spend a significant part of their careers in the military. To join the Army, Navy, or

Air Force, you must be a U.S. citizen, at least board-eligible in your specialty, physically fit according to military standards, and under 42 years of age. There are on-going shortages of general surgeons, orthopaedic surgeons, otolaryngologists, family physicians, and obstetricians who are needed to serve military personnel and their dependents at bases around the world. You may also apply to work part-time in the Army National Guard one weekend per month and two weeks annually. You may also be called for active duty in times of national emergencies. Benefits include a substantial sign-on bonus, repayment of certain types of school loans, and a supplemental paycheck to your regular non-military income.

Occupational Medicine. See Part II of the book for the chapter "Occupational Medicine."

Prison Health Care. Many physicians who are employed in this field have a strong commitment to the care of the medically underserved. Having foreign language skills is helpful in this setting. You could be employed by a city, state, or federal agency, depending upon the prison site. A female physician who was the medical director at a women's prison says that "women are tremendously neglected inside the prison, and that's not even taking into account the gynecologic issues."[13] In addition, there is a growing geriatric population in prisons. Most prison physicians have a background in family medicine, internal medicine, or emergency medicine. There is an orientation towards chronic care in state and federal prisons because the average stay is long. The Society of Correctional Physicians has a goal of establishing a recognized specialty in correctional medicine. The general preventive medicine residency at the University of Texas in Galveston, Texas has a focus on this area.[14]

School Health. Student health centers exist on all U.S. university campuses and residential high schools. They primarily serve a combination of students, staff, faculty, and their dependents. Their mission may range from first aid and emergency care to a more comprehensive health care system. They are staffed by a team of health care professionals, may be open 24 hours a day, and even have infirmary beds. Some smaller campuses contract with local physicians to supplement non-physician care offered at the student health center. Mental health services may be offered outside of the student health center. Student health physicians earn less than in other settings with a median salary of $91,000 for family physicians, but many accept it for the lifestyle it offers. A doctor typically works an eight-hour daytime shift and perhaps weekends with no call. Malpractice insurance is paid and there is generous vacation time. Some campuses offer tuition reimbursement for family members.[15]

NON-CLINICAL PATHWAYS

Administrative Medicine. See Part 3 of the book for the chapter on "Administrative Medicine."

Broadcasting and Movies. Your local news program will most likely have a regular health segment presented by a physician. Consumer interest in health news is high, and radio and television stations are eager to accommodate their listening public. The AMA offers training in working in the broadcasting field. A broad-based medical training and practice background is advantageous because you will need to discuss a wide variety of medical topics. Although few physicians will make this a full-time career, some have, such as Doctors Art Ulene and Dean Edell.

Television shows and movies employ physicians as technical advisors. For example, the television show *ER* had a number of physicians involved in its creation. Neal Baer, MD, the supervising producer and one of the writers, attended film school prior to medical school and was an intern in pediatrics, working during *ER* hiatuses.[16]

Insurance Medicine. With the growth of managed care, physicians are sought in the insurance industry. In addition to the traditional role of a life insurance medical director who advises underwriters in risk selection and examination requirements for applicants, physicians can consult with claim examiners and work with lawyers to interpret the wording of policies. A broad specialty, such as family medicine or internal medicine, is most desirable.[17] For more information on a closely related career path, see the chapter on "Administrative Medicine."

Journalism and Writing. Many physicians begin their writing careers while in medical school or residency, often because they need to share their experiences with others. It is possible to blend the two careers, especially if you have chosen a specialty that has opportunities for part-time employment. One internist who practices occupational medicine tells that he averages approximately 20 hours of clinical work a week and spends the rest of his time writing on medical topics for the public. He believes that "research for my writing has made me a better doctor."[18] You might serve as a part- or full-time consultant to a publisher of medical books or be an editor for a magazine, medical journal, or newsletter.

Journalists writing on health care issues are finding expanding job opportunities as the public desires more information. There is an opportunity for physicians in smaller communities to write health news for local newspapers, but a wider audience is needed to make it a full-time career. Non-physician writers dominate the field, with only 12.5 percent of the members of the American Medical Writers Association possessing a medical degree. Even with the advantages of understanding medical terminology and having clinical experience, the successful physician in this field must be able to explain medical phenomena clearly and have a passion for writing.[19]

Legal Medicine. The American College of Legal Medicine has 1,100 members —professionals who have both law and medicine degrees. Some medical schools offer joint MD/JD programs.[20] Your career path is dependent upon your medical specialty training. A variety of clinical specialties, especially surgery, family medicine, and internal medicine, can prepare you to represent either plaintiffs or defendants in malpractice suits. A neurosurgeon has turned his sights on lawsuits against HMOs. A radiation oncologist consultant describes being on a law school faculty, teaching health law and law and bioethics.[20]

Organized Medicine. This is the most common expression of physician volunteer involvement as individuals serve on committees and task forces of the AMA, the state and local medical societies, and the multitude of specialty societies. However, a few physicians devote their careers to organized medicine full time, serving as executive directors of their chosen specialty's major medical organizations.

Public Service. Relatively few physicians choose full-time public service. Some will become health policy analysts and researchers in government or academia. Others will enter politics and become candidates for public office. When elected, these physicians tend to focus on health related legislation. For example, John Kitzhaber, MD, governor of Oregon, designed the Oregon Health Plan, and Howard Dean, MD, governor of Vermont, created a program that provides health insurance to low-income children. The former is an emergency medicine physician; the latter, an internist.

Research. A physician researcher may be employed by an academic institution, the federal government, or a pharmaceutical firm. A total of 14,087 physicians are engaged in this activity according to the AMA.

In academics, dual MD and PhD degrees are valuable. The training in these combined-degree programs lasts 7 to 8 years—4 years of medical school and 3 to 4 years of PhD work. Most graduates enter residency training, primarily in internal medicine, pediatrics, pathology, and surgery.[21]

Researchers work for the federal government in a variety of agencies including the Alcohol, Drug Abuse, and Mental Health Administration; the Centers for Disease Control (CDC); the Food and Drug Administration (FDA); and the National Institutes of Health (NIH). Dual MD and MPH degrees are desirable for employment at the CDC and other government health-policy agencies. For clinical research, dual MD and PhD degrees are an asset.

Pharmaceutical companies recruit mainly subspecialty internal medicine physicians to work in research efforts involving "designing new studies, writing protocols, initiating and monitoring studies, interpreting data, preparing medical reports, extrapolating results, and developing a clinical strategy to bring a new drug or a new indication for an existing drug forward."[22] You can expect to earn $110,000 to $120,000 plus benefits and bonuses in an entry-level position. Experience in patient care and an extensive background in anatomy and physiology are valuable assets in securing employment in this competitive field.

Special Niches. There are a variety of other opportunities that are possible to pursue that blend your own personal talents and interests with medicine. Often these other interests pre-date your interest in medicine.

Financially astute physicians might consider a career as a health care stock portfolio manager or a pharmaceutical industry analyst, in which they use their scientific knowledge to evaluate new products.

Because he held masters degrees in bioengineering and business administration before entering medical school, one physician developed his own medical device and software development company. As a practicing internist, he finds that patients' needs often "inspire" his engineering.[18]

GEOGRAPHIC LOCATION
Urban Versus Rural

Your geographic location will be determined to some degree by your specialty. Neurosurgeons and other tertiary-care physicians need to practice in major urban centers to have a large enough patient base. Primary and some secondary care physicians, such as general surgeons and psychiatrists, can practice in both large and small communities. Primary care physicians have the most choice of where to practice. Research has shown that men are more likely than women to practice in rural areas.[23] Unrepresented minority physician status is an important factor in the choice of an inner-city practice.[23]

Your perceptions of the advantages of an urban or rural practice for you and loved ones in your life may outweigh your specialty preference. The employment market in a rural location may be too limited for your partner. The fast pace and relative anonymity of a city may not appeal to you. Small town schools may not offer advanced classes for your children; city crime may be seen as a threat to your personal safety.

Selected Geographic Options

International Medicine. You may have entered medical school committed to a full-time career in international health. More likely, you have a strong interest in serving overseas either for a few years after completing your residency training or for short-term experiences throughout your practice years. You may be motivated by a desire to serve or by the adventure of travel.

You can engage in clinical service in missionary hospitals or clinics, most of which are located in underdeveloped parts of South America, Asia, and Africa. Most expenses are the responsibility of the physician unless you are directing or developing the program. There are even three Mercy Ships, sponsored by a national Christian organization, that serve as floating hospitals.[24] Assignments can last for months or years. You can even serve for a few days, such as when responding to natural disasters with a medical relief agency. Doctors Without Borders, one of the largest nonprofit medical relief groups with a primary focus on emergency missions, has over 2000 doctors, nurses, and other medical professionals currently volunteering in over 70 countries. Most programs, however, prefer at least a six-month commitment, although surgeons and anesthesiologists are recruited for stays as short as six weeks.[25] The specialties most needed are those that do not rely on high technology—family medicine, internal medicine, and pediatrics. Surgeons are valued greatly, especially if they are comfortable with rudimentary resources and are proficient in general surgery, urology, orthopaedics, and gynecology. Pregnancy-related operations, groin hernia procedures, and appendectomies are common, as are fracture care and urologic procedures. The surgeons who can bring equipment and set up temporary facilities, such as ophthalmologists and otolaryngologists, also are greatly needed.

You might also serve abroad as a public health and preventive medicine officer. One physician who has served internationally as a public health officer since 1960 says that there is currently "great demand for physicians with a masters degree in public health or special skills in maternal and child health, health education, health planning and management and, of course, special training in HIV/STDs." He advocates having language skills, citing the benefits of his knowledge of French in Cambodia and a number of African countries.[26]

In addition to superior medical knowledge and diagnostic skills, an understanding of and sensitivity to the local culture is essential. Working with local support personnel may require patience and flexibility. Needed medical supplies often are unavailable, and electricity and hot running water are not always reliable.

The American Medical Student Association (AMSA) and the American Academy of Family Physicians publish listings of international medical opportunities for medical students and physicians.

Cruise Medicine. For those who seek part-time travel as a component of their careers, there is cruise medicine. Newer ships resemble small cities and can accommodate as many as 6000 passengers plus crewmembers whose medical problems can range from seasickness to a life-or-death illness. Most sought are physicians who have broad-based skills, such as family medicine or emergency medicine physicians, but who also have some expertise in surgery and cardiology. The number of medical personnel on board varies with the size of the ship; a physician's compensation is set by the cruise company. While on board, the physician has set office hours, but is "on call" 24 hours a day. Most contracts are short—two or three weeks—because there is a preference for physicians who are engaged in active practices.[27]

Tropical, Travel, and Wilderness Medicine. The discipline of tropical medicine, originally focused on the health of civil servants, merchants, military personnel, missionaries, and selected indigenous populations, has evolved to include a broader scope of concerns. The emphasis is on the health status of populations (rather than special groups) who reside in tropical and developing countries. Chief among these concerns is the treatment and control of infectious diseases, especially with airline travel making the world smaller and more vulnerable to an unexpected epidemic.

A related area is travel medicine (emporiatrics), a field that includes physicians trained in tropical, occupational, and internal medicine as well as family medicine. The emphasis is on promoting the health of those who travel. You might be in a full-time research career, serve as staff in a health department or travel clinic, or be on the faculty at one of the seven academic institutions offering course work in tropical medicine. The American Society of Tropical Medicine and Hygiene sponsors an examination for Certification in Clinical Tropical Medicine and Travelers Health. Prerequisites are completion of a society-approved course of study in tropical medicine and at least two months overseas clinical experience.[28]

A newer focus is wilderness medicine, which is the practice of medicine in remote locations and extreme environments. One physician describes it as "off-the-beaten-path" medicine. It contains elements of rural, emergency, and sports medicine. A broad-based residency would prepare you for this type of career path. Opportunities for full-time employment exist at national park clinics or in related research. Most physicians, however, engage in wilderness medicine activities part time, perhaps leading rafting and mountaineering expeditions or seasonally staffing remote medical clinics.

Topics at a recent Wilderness Medical Society (WMS) "Travel and Environmental Medicine Course" included "Immunization Update," "Medical Kits for Travelers," and "Acute Diarrhea in the Returned Traveler," topics helpful to the physician who incorporates travel medicine into his or her medical practice. In addition, there were sessions on "Emerging Third-World Diseases of Concern," "Improvising Medical Solutions in the Field," and "Special Medical Considerations in Long-Term Travelers and Expatriates," topics of greater interest to physicians and health professionals practicing in remote sites. Another wilderness medicine conference offered workshops on "Orienteering/Routefinding (Mountain Navigation)," "Frostbite Update," and "Wild Animal Attacks." The more than 3000 WMS members share a common interest in backpacking, traveling, skiing, and diving as well as conservation and medical concerns.

Locum Tenens. All specialties are recruited for work as a "locum tenens." You are hired to take the place of a physician who is temporarily absent. The position may last from several days to months. The compensation varies according to your specialty and the geographic location. Primary care salaries are approximately $300 a day. New graduates often sign up as "locum tenens" physicians to try out practice styles and locations. There is even a journal, Locus Life, that is "dedicated to locum tenens physicians" and offers a free online subscription to physicians.

LOOKING AHEAD

No matter where you choose to live and what practice option you follow, your medical career ideally should develop over the years to match your personal interests. You will be involved in assessing and reassessing your choices, hopefully with the aid of family members and professional colleagues. In the final analysis, however, your specialty choice should reflect your personal values.

REFERENCES

1. Aronson SM. Physicians and students who abandon medical careers often move on to achieve greatness in other professions. *Fam Phys Recruiter* (Western Ed.), September 1998, pp. 1, 20.
2. Fraker S. Physicians enter the job market. *JAMA* 1998;279(17):1399.
3. Frieden J. Two boards join to offer hospitalist certification. *Fam Pract News* November 15, 2009; p.62.
4. Press release. MGMA/SHM Survey Report shows that compensation model affects hospitalist productivity and salary. September 9, 2010. www.hospitalmedicine.org accessed January 15, 2011.
5. Wachter RM, Goldman L. The emerging role of "hospitalists" in the American health care system. *N Engl J Med* 1996;335(7):514–516.
6. Daily L. Demand for new specialties. *Phys Finan News* 1998;16(2):S25.
7. Flanders S. A watershed moment. *The Hospitalist* December 2009; p. 48.
8. Greene K. Physicians revive house calls, lured by Medicare fees. *Wall Street Journal*, August 2, 200; pp. B 1 & 4.
9. Binius T. Return of the house call. *Am Med News* 1999;43 (2):29-31.
10. Thoren H. Performing arts medicine gaining a larger audience. *Fam Pract News* 1992;22(18):18.

11. Siwek J. Quoted in *AAFP Reporter.* February 1991, p. 7.
12. Delmar D. Emphasis for academic practice shifting from research to clinical. *Phys Finan News* 1995;13(10):S9.
13. Zeitlin A. Volunteering behind bars. *Diversion* 1998;25(5):35–40.
14. Kirkwood J. Prisoner patients. *Unique Opportunities 2002;12(4):40-48.*
15. Steinberg C. Ivy-covered practice: college health doctors trade pay for lifestyle. Phys Finan News 2000; 18(12):1 & 25.
16. O'Connor MM. An interview with Neal Baer, MD, the doctor behind *ER. JAMA* 1998;280(9):855.
17. Steinberg C. Insurance industry offers opportunities for doctors to impact medical practice. *Phys Finan News* 1994;12(3):S14.
18. Moskow S. Double vision. *Am Med News* 1995;35(2):21,29.
19. Taylor RB. Medical writing: A guide for clinicians, educators and researchers. New York: Springer; 2011.
20. Daily L. Wide variety of career paths open to physician/attorneys. *Phys Finan News* 1998;16(2):30.
21. Schwartz P, Gaulton GN. Addressing the needs of basic and clinical research: Analysis of the University of Pennsylvania MD-PhD program graduates. *JAMA* 1999; 281(1):96–99.
22. Timpane J. Everywhere and then some: Physicians making careers in biopharmaceuticals. *JAMA* 1998;279(17):1401.
23. Xu G, Veloski JJ, Hojat M, Politzer RM, Rabinowitz HK, Rattner S. Factors influencing physicians' choices to practice in inner-city or rural areas. *Acad Med* 1997;72(12):1026.
24. Spencer M. Mercy ships, ahoy. *Diversion* 1998;26(2):226–231.
25. Stevens S. A wide world of opportunities exist for international relief volunteers. *Phys Finan News* 1997;15(16):S8–10.
26. Montague J. Public health physicians needed overseas. Letters. *Unique Opportunities,* July/August 1997, p. 58.
27. Korcok M. Maritime experts urge examination of shipboard medical services. *Am Med News* 1990;29:3,38–39.
28. Exam to certify knowledge in tropical medicine. *Am Med News* 1996;39(24):42.

PART 5

AFTER YOU HAVE CHOSEN A SPECIALTY

Planning for Residency Choice

"All of a sudden it was July, and a single burning thought struck fear into the hearts of all fourth-year students— finding the perfect residency. One minute we are studying general pathology and physical diagnosis; the next minute we have to decide what type of medicine to practice and where to do a residency. To compound the problem, even if one makes careful decisions about a specialty and residency program, it is becoming more and more difficult to "match" at a favorite residency program."[1]

—Billy Katibah, fourth year medical student

MATCHING FOR A RESIDENCY POSITION IS AN ADMISSIONS process like any other admissions process: you send for information, choose where to apply, fill in application forms, go for interviews, and select your choices. What distinguishes it from other admissions procedures is the relative lack of information you have until the end of your third year of medical school and the large number of rumors about the "Match." This chapter should help you sort out "fact" from "fiction" by answering some common questions about matching programs.

THE MATCHING PROCESS

The National Resident Matching Program

Most medical students find a residency position through the National Resident Matching Program (NRMP; Internet address: www.aamc. org/nrmp), a service that, since 1952, has been facilitating student and program matches and announcing the results on a uniform date and time. The NRMP was initiated in an era when internship positions outnumbered graduating students two to one and students found that they were being pressured to accept appointments early in their fourth year from less competitive programs while awaiting decisions from more favored residencies. The differences in appointment dates among programs left the decision whether to accept or to wait and hope for a better offer entirely up to the student.

Today, a computer makes the decision—in less than three minutes—but your planning probably has started months or (hopefully) years before. You should refer to the suggested timetable in Part 1 for tasks to be accomplished in preparation for specialty selection and residency application.

Who Should Participate in the NRMP?

All students should participate in the NRMP, including those who are applying to military and advanced specialty programs that operate their own matches. If you do not match in one of the other matches, you still will be eligible to secure a residency position through the NRMP.

Matching opportunities for shared-schedule positions and couples are offered through the NRMP. These are discussed later in this Part of the book.

Medical schools may sponsor former graduates from their institution who deferred application to residency at the time of their graduation. However, students and graduates of Canadian medical schools and schools accredited by the American Osteopathic Association must register as Independent Applicants. Also included in this category are graduates of non-United States unaccredited medical schools who hold an unrestricted license to practice medicine in the United States or who have passed the necessary examinations offered by the Educational Commission for Foreign Medical Graduates.

What Are the Programs Within the NRMP?

Virtually all civilian first-year postgraduate programs in family medicine, general surgery, internal medicine, obstetrics-gynecology, pathology, and pediatrics, and most of the first-year positions in psychiatry and emergency medicine are offered as *Categorical (C) positions* in the NRMP. You can enter these programs with no previous residency training and complete all the necessary requirements for that specialty.

Primary Care (M) positions are categorical primary care or generalist positions offered in some internal medicine and pediatric residency programs.

All *Transitional (P) positions* are offered through the NRMP. These are in a first-year program that offers training in several specialties prior to your applying for a second year in a specific specialty. You may have rotations in surgery, internal medicine, pediatrics, emergency medicine, obstetrics-gynecology, and psychiatry during this year. Be aware, however, that most surgical specialties, family medicine, internal medicine, and pediatrics will not give you full credit for this year of training, and you may have to repeat part or all of your internship year.

Some programs in anesthesiology, dermatology, neurological surgery, neurology, nuclear medicine, ophthalmology, orthopaedic surgery, otolaryngology, physical medicine and rehabilitation, psychiatry, diagnostic radiology, radiation oncology, and urology offer *Preliminary (P) positions* in internal medicine, pediatrics, and general surgery for one or two years prior to entering training in their specialties. This is essentially the same program as a categorical internship year in internal medicine or general surgery, and, if you choose to continue in one of these specialties, will be counted as a full year of training.

There are also *Advanced (A) positions* participating in the NRMP. These programs require one or more years of preliminary training in internal medicine, pediatrics, or surgery, or a transitional internship year, but you can apply to them as a senior medical student. Some institutions arrange for preliminary positions for all who are accepted into their advanced specialty programs; others do not. You may have to complete two applications: one for the *Advanced positions* and one for the preliminary years.

The NRMP offers *Physician (R) positions* starting in the year of the Match for those physicians who have already completed some residency training. These positions are not available to senior U.S. medical students.

There are also *Fellowship Positions* for those who have completed a residency and wish to subspecialize further. The Medical Specialties Matching Program (MSMP) currently offers positions in all the internal medicine subspecialties described in Part 2 of this book. In addition, there are numerous other subspecialty matches managed by the NRMP (see www.nrmp.org/fellow/index/html for the full listing).

Another option for residency is the *Combined Training Programs* that lead to Board certification in more than one field. These programs are detailed in individual specialty chapters earlier in this book, and a complete listing is found in the American Medical Association Fellowship and Residency Electronic Interactive Database Access System (AMA-FREIDA). The table below details the combined programs.

Combined Residencies	Number of Programs	Number of First Year Positions
Internal Medicine/Dermatology	8	6
Internal Medicine/Emergency Medicine	12	24
Internal Medicine/Family Medicine	2	6
Internal Medicine/Medical Genetics	4	2
Internal Medicine/Neurology	6	2

Combined Residencies	Number of Programs	Number of First Year Positions
Internal Medicine/Pediatrics	81	359
Internal Medicine/Preventive Medicine	8	7
Internal Medicine/Psychiatry	16	20

When Do I Apply to the NRMP?

Assuming you have decided on a specialty, you need to find out whether the specialty has its own match outside the NRMP (currently, child neurology, ophthalmology, plastic surgery and urology), whether some programs in your chosen specialty are in the NRMP and some are not (some programs in anesthesiology, orthopaedic surgery, and otolaryngology), or if all the programs participate fully in the NRMP. Each option will involve different timetables because the military and some specialties match earlier.

You need to register and "sign' the agreement on-line, and it must be submitted by November 30. Your school's Dean's office verifies that you are eligible to participate in the Match once you have applied. Your agreement must be accompanied by a nonrefundable application fee that allows you to rank ten hospitals on your rank order list; if you wish to rank more, there will be an additional fee for each.

What Are My Obligations by Participating in the NRMP?

If you participate in the NRMP process through Match Day, you are obligated to accept the position that is offered to you. However, if you are accepted at a military or advanced specialty program, you can withdraw from the NRMP.

If you are participating in both the Canadian Resident Matching Service (CaRMS) and the NRMP, you will be expected to accept a position if matched into the Canadian Program, which has an earlier schedule for matching than the NRMP. The CaRMS will inform the NRMP that you have matched, and your name will be deleted from the NRMP match.

Other Matching Programs

The US Armed Forces Match. Medical students who are members of the Army, Navy, or Air Force programs participate in a separate match for residency positions in the military programs (military programs are discussed in a later section).

Advanced Specialty Programs With Their Own Matching Programs. Some specialties have matching programs for residency positions at the second or later years outside of the NRMP. At present, most or all of the programs in ophthalmology and plastic surgery participate in the San Francisco Matching Program, P.O. Box 7584, San Francisco, CA 94120. Telephone: (415) 447-0350. Internet address: www. SFMATCH.org. Urology match information can be obtained from the American Urological Association Residency Matching Program, 2425 West Loop South, Suite 333, Houston, TX 77027. Internet address: www. auanet.org.

These matches are conducted earlier than the NRMP and you will be required to register with the NRMP for the required preliminary training (for example, one or two years of general surgery prior to otolaryngology).

Nonmatch Programs. A direct application process is currently used by most programs in preventive medicine, nuclear medicine, and a few programs in psychiatry. Also, you will need to apply directly to newly approved programs that are not yet listed in a match program.

Osteopathic Programs. Osteopathic medical students apply to the Intern/Resident Registration Program (the "AOA" Match) conducted by the National Matching Services, Inc. on behalf of the American Osteopathic Association (AOA). However, not all students participate. Those with military commitments participate in the military matching program (see later chapter in this Part of the book). There are declining numbers of funded osteopathic internship positions and increasing numbers of osteopathic graduates. As a result, about half of the osteo-pathic graduates enter accredited osteopathic residencies. Since 1985, a residency program can be dual-accredited by both the ACGME and the AOA. The topic of dual-accreditation is controversial. Since 2001, a Doctor of Osteopathy resident in any MD residency program can apply for osteopathic approval of their training, but MDs are generally not permitted to train in osteopathic (AOA-accredited) residencies, although this is being studied.[3-5]

There are osteopathic residencies in a large number of specialty areas, and they are listed annually on the *AOA Opportunities database*. Applicants register with the Electronic Residency Application Service (ERAS) to apply to programs. The Match results are released in February, a month earlier than the NRMP.

Part-Time and Shared-Schedule Positions

Part-time and shared-schedule residency positions have existed since the 1960s. They are of interest to an individual who wishes to extend his or her residency beyond the usual length (four years rather than the customary three years of a family medicine, internal medicine or pediatrics residency) or two persons sharing a single residency position, each working a reduced schedule over a proportionately longer period of time. An applicant may negotiate a part-time or shared contract with any residency program. Previously, residencies in the primary care specialties (family medicine, internal medicine, obstetrics-gynecology, and pediatrics) were required to offer a shared position if they received federal monies and admitted 12 or more residents per year. This law was repealed in August 1981.[6]

For a shared residency, the partners enroll individually in the NRMP and submit a "shared residency pair form" (available from your medical school or the NRMP), which assigns the pair one match number and one name, e.g., "Smith/Jones Ann/Michael." The pair submits one rank order list that they agree on. The program ranks the pair by their "name" and number just as they would individuals who are doing "solo" residencies.

Common Arrangements for Shared-Schedule Residencies[*]

Interdigitating Format. The residents are on the same clinical services together, and care for the same patients simultaneously. Through

---

[*] Modification of an article originally published in the Dual Doctor Families Newsletter 1983;2(1):1,6–7. Used with permission.

careful communication and cooperation they take turns with call, chasing down lab results, and managing patients. They probably will stay on a particular ward service several weeks or months longer than their colleagues in order to achieve the same level of experience. However, they also should be able to take alternating afternoons off. They may take their vacations separately or together. They are collectively responsible to their supervisors. This plan is job-sharing in the true sense of the word!

Alternating Format. One resident works while the other one is off. The "on" resident works full-time and keeps the same hours as colleagues on the ward team. Meanwhile the partner enjoys the benefits of being off. It is possible in some residencies offering shared positions to work more than half-time under this format and to finish proportionately sooner. In certain residencies, including all family medicine programs, the off-resident is required to return several half-days per week to provide continuing care for his or her patients. Thus, in the alternating format, the "off" person may want or be required to attend to the ongoing care of patients.

Salary Arrangements. Anything is possible; negotiate and then get it in writing. According to the repealed federal law, a shared resident was to work at least two-thirds time for at least half-pay and full benefits. Some argue that a person should receive pay in direct proportion to hours worked. Others argue that a resident should pay extra for the privilege of not working as much as other colleagues and that because a residency program is inconvenienced in order to coordinate the shared-pair's schedules, the program is therefore entitled to more "doctor per dollar." In addition, many programs do not have the dollars to pay a shared-resident pair more than one full salary.

Strategies for Applying and Interviewing. Rule number one is: have your act together! To propose a part-time or shared-schedule residency position, you will need to be able to state your reasons. A common reason to work part-time or share a residency involves family responsibilities. Other people may want time to do research, to pursue a second profession simultaneously, to reduce stress, to increase recreational opportunities, or to "be a whole person and not just a doctor."

For a shared-schedule position, decide carefully what you want your shared residency to be like and write a concise plan. A written agreement between the co-applicants detailing their goals and aspirations is wise. When you apply, each applicant must fill out a separate application and obtain a separate dean's letter. Consider the benefits and disadvantages of discussing the shared-residency proposal in your personal statement and of having the writers of your letters of recommendation support your plan. Remember that in addition to selling your proposal as a good and practical idea, you must also convince them that you are individually better-than-average for their program.

Before an interview is arranged, try to "feel the program out" about your proposal. You may waste time and money going where a part-time or shared-schedule residency is not workable. For a shared-schedule residency, arrange interviews on the same day and, if possible, try to arrange at least one joint interview with a powerful person, ideally the residency director, so you can discuss the proposal together. Both applicants should contribute to the discussion equally and should complement each other's remarks. Do not be surprised if the interviewer has never heard of a shared residency. Memorize a brief outline of the important points of your proposal. The interviewer will be impressed that the "team" is organized, and time will be saved by not having to hear two similar versions. Be sure to talk to current residents about the program and your proposal, and ask if it sounds feasible. Get detailed information about the residency's scheduled rotations so that after the interview, you can design and submit a sample shared schedule to fit their program. Be willing to be flexible about scheduling if your plan does not quite fit what they think they can offer. At some point, they must have your proposal in writing. It never hurts to remind them about the match rules for shared applicants one more time just before you expect them to fill out their rank order form. You wouldn't want to risk not being ranked simply because they didn't remember how to do it.

Programs offering shared-schedule positions are identified in the AMA-FREIDA computer system and should be contacted directly. A national survey of pediatric residency programs[8] reported that 24 percent of 190 programs on AMA-FRIEDA indicated that they offer part-time and/or shared residency positions, but only a few residents held such positions during a 3-year period.

Larger programs were more likely to offer such positions and most of them are in family medicine, internal medicine, pediatrics, psychiatry, and child psychiatry.

SEEKING INFORMATION

Gather information as early as possible on both the process of applying to residency and details on the residency programs in your chosen specialty. The premier website resource on both choosing a specialty and applying to residency is the Association of American Medical Colleges' Careers in Medicine site, www.aamc.org/cim.

In addition, you should go directly to the residency program's website and the website of the major organization for the specialty (listed at the end of each chapter in Part 2 of this book). Most specialty societies have posted listings of residency programs in their specialty on their websites.

For a complete listing of all residency programs, there is the annually updated computer program known as AMA-FREIDA (https://freida.ama-assn.org/Freida/user/viewProgramSearch.do)   for which each residency program is asked to provide information on over 100 items, including: characteristics of residents and faculty; call schedules; benefits provided; curriculum; availability of "shared-schedule positions"; and name, address, and telephone number of the program director.

The American Medical Student Association (AMSA; Internet address: www.amsa.org) offers the *Student Guide to the Appraisal and Selection of House Staff Training Programs;* this is a valuable resource that offers advice on resumes, letters of recommendation, interviewing, and evaluation of residency programs.

Resources at your school—graduating seniors and residents—can offer opinions on various programs, some of which will be subjective. A career counseling service may provide evaluations from alumni, a library of brochures and directories, and personal counseling. Websites are sources of information about specific residencies with reviews written by both applicants and residents in the programs. Look at the websites for Student Doctor Network and Scutwork.com listed in the Appendix of this book.

APPLYING TO RESIDENCIES

What Should I Know About Filling Out My Residency Program Applications?

Applications vary in format and information requested; you will need plenty of time to complete them. Students use the Electronic Residency Application Service (ERAS) at www.aamc.org/eras to apply. The application fee for up to 10 programs is $75; 11–20 programs, $8 each; 21–30 programs, $15 each; above 30 programs, $25 each.

Here are some tips:

Your curriculum vitae and personal statement should be thorough but concise, allowing the reader to learn about your most favorable qualities and achievements. Be sure to emphasize areas of common interest; for example, if a program is located in a city where you have family members or if you have participated in activities such as research or community service that are pertinent to that program's focus of interest.

Your Medical School Performance Report, (formerly called the Dean's Letter), may be written by the Dean of Student Affairs alone or in conjunction with a clinical advisor. It will be based primarily on your grades and clerkship performance with a stated purpose "... as an evaluation of a medical student's performance (rather than a recommendation or prediction of future performance)."[7] Some specialties will weigh grades more heavily than others, but I cannot emphasize too strongly the increasing importance of grades, especially those in the clinical rotation of your chosen specialty, but also, for some specialties, those from the first two years of medical school. This letter will also provide personal bibliographic data; the key feature is that most letters have a final sentence that gives a summary evaluation of you as an applicant relative to your peers.

Request a letter of recommendation from at least one physician faculty member in your chosen specialty. Other letters should come from faculty members who know you well and who can write enthusiastically about your abilities. If you approach someone who hesitates about writing your letter, do not press the matter—ask someone else. If a faculty member has a connection with a program that interests you, that is an added bonus—"old school ties" are very helpful.

When your application is completed, submit it. The sooner it arrives, the sooner you can be invited to schedule an interview. It is possible that the more competitive programs will have full interview schedules if you wait too long. It is especially important to plan ahead if you are trying to coordinate interviews at a number of nearby programs.

Be sure to keep a record of all your applications, including photocopies of correspondence and notes on telephone conversations. As you start to schedule visits to programs, names and dates will start to accumulate and an organized record keeping system is most helpful.

What Advice Can You Offer About Interviewing?

The interview may be the most important part of the application process—both for you and for the program. There is an old saying: your record gets you the interview; your interview gets you the job. It is not only a chance for the program to evaluate you, but an opportunity for you to evaluate the program, the hospital, and the geographic location. Some programs interview all applicants; others select those they will interview on the basis of grades and National Board scores. Most students interview in November, December, and January of their fourth year. Your spouse or significant other should be included in this process, if not by actually accompanying you as you interview, then at least being involved in the post-interview evaluation of programs and their geographic locations.

You will have many questions, but first read the program material so you do not ask what is already provided. Be sure to talk to residents currently in the program—they will probably be your best source of information. You will find suggestions on questions to ask in the AMSA *Student Guide to the Appraisal and Selection of House Staff*

Training Programs, Iserson's *Getting Into a Residency*, and Katta and Desai's *The Successful Match.*

Try not to schedule your interviews too close together—you will find that you need time to assess what you have seen before jumping into the next interview. If this is not possible, keep as many notes as possible—even though it seems you could not forget how unhappy the residents were at a program, two weeks later you may find yourself wondering which program it was.

You may be asked by an interviewer how you plan to rank the program; this is acceptable. However, verbal agreements are not binding and should not influence your ranking of programs. Some unmatched students have discovered this sad fact too late.

After the interview you may be sufficiently impressed with a program to write a letter indicating so. This is perfectly acceptable – send the letter to the program director if you met him or her and to the faulty who interviewed you. Also, write a note to thank the administrative assistant/residency coordinator who does the behind the scenes work to make the interviews runs smoothly. Personalize each letter, either referring to something you discussed in your interview or something specific about how you feel the you would be a good match for the program.

If you decide not to keep an interview appointment or, for some reason, cannot get there, call as soon as possible so that another applicant can interview in your time slot. If possible, you will be given consideration for rescheduling. Remember, if you are unmatched, you may wish to make contact with this program if they have an open position.

How Should I Rank My Choices?

Students spend a great deal of time discussing various strategies—all supposedly guaranteed to secure your first choice program. The rank order list is confidential for both the student and the program and must be submitted by both to the NRMP before the end of February. The student's wishes are the basis upon which the computer makes close choices; that is, the program is tilted in the student's favor. Therefore, what you want most should go to the top of your list. You can list more than one specialty on your rank order list, and this may be wise if you are applying for a highly competitive field of medicine. Most of all, you need to include a spectrum of programs: those that may be too competitive but are most desirable; those that are realistic and acceptable; and those that are even below your abilities, but are also acceptable. It is probably better to go unmatched than to list unacceptable programs just to be safe. For further information, see the chapter on What Happens If You Don't Match.

REFERENCES

1. Katibah B. Student newsletter. *Tar Heel Practitioner,* September–October 1983, p. 12.
2. www.nrmp.org/about_nrmp/new_policies.html.,accessed September 14, 2002.
3. http://en.wikipedia.org/wiki/ Comparison_of_MD_and_DO_in_ the_United_Statesaccessed January 6, 2011.
4. Schierhorn C. Educators at summit frame future of Osteopathic Graduate Medical Education. *The DO magazine.* American Osteopathic Association. June 2008. p.22-27
5. Schierhorn C. Slumping Osteopathic Graduate Medical Education piques educators at summit. *The D.O. magazine.* American Osteopathic Association. Feb 2008. p.22-28
6. Carling PC, Hayward K, Coakley EH, Wolf AMD. Part-time residency training in internal medicine: Analysis of a ten -year experience. *Acad Med* 1999;74(3):282–284.
7. A Guide to the Preparation of the Medical Student Performance Evaluation. Association of American Medical Colleges, 2002.
8. Holmes AV, Cuff WL, Socolar RR. Part-time residency in pediatrics: Description of current practice. *Pediatrics* July 2005; 116(1):32-37.

Military Programs

INFORMATION IN THIS CHAPTER IS BASED ON INTERVIEWS
with medical students and physicians who are members of the Armed
Forces Health Professions Scholarship Program (HPSP) in the Air
Force, Army, or Navy. Devon Greer, MS 4, who has an Navy Health
Professions Scholarship; Brittany Millard-Hasting, who has an Air
Force Health Professions Scholarship; and Jesse Schonau-Taylor, MS
4, who has an Army Health Professions Scholarship at the Oregon
Health & Science University School of Medicine, reviewed and
updated this chapter for this current edition of the book.

WHY SHOULD SOMEONE CONSIDER APPLYING TO THE ARMED FORCES HEALTH PROFESSIONS SCHOLARSHIP PROGRAM?

The Armed Forces HPSP offers scholarships to medical students who
are willing to serve in the active duty military. Financial and personal
benefits vary with the individual's needs, desires, and philosophy, but
there is a consensus among student respondents that money is a prime
factor: "It offers good benefits without loan obligations," "It elim-
inates money as a consideration for specialty choice," and "A military
residency pays more than civilian residencies." Specifically, the
program pays for full tuition, required books, Licensure examinations,
nonexpendable equipment and most academic fees, a monthly stipend

for $10^1/_2$ months of each school year, and full pay and allowances of a second lieutenant or ensign for the remaining $1^1/_2$ months of each medical school year.

Additionally, as career physicians in the military, you do not have to worry about paying for your malpractice insurance. The base pay for military physicians is based on rank and time in service, with modest additional pay provided for specialty training.

One student said, "the military offers opportunities that civilian medicine rarely offers such as flight medicine, undersea/dive medicine and general medical officer. These were my main reasons for joining."

WHAT ARE THE RESPONSIBILITIES AND COMMITMENTS ONCE A MILITARY SCHOLARSHIP IS ACCEPTED?

You are obligated after internship, residency, or fellowship program to one year of active duty service for each year of medical school financed, with a minimum of three years obligation. Also, you are required to engage in six weeks of active duty training during each school year. This usually involves a medical rotation at a military hospital for which you receive academic credit.

Traditionally, the scholarship recipient will complete their service's officer training school in the summer between the first and second years of the scholarship. This fulfills one of the six-week training obligations. However, it is possible to complete service's officer training school before starting your first year of medical school. This would allow you to use your summer between first and second year to be in a health related experience and not training. The other six-week requirement is usually completed as a four-week clerkship in the fourth year of medical school, with the remaining two weeks spent at home.

WHO CAN PARTICIPATE IN THE MILITARY RESIDENCY MATCH?

First-year positions in military residencies are required of those who are graduates of the Uniformed Services University of the Health

Sciences (USUHS) and are competitive for those who have participated in the HPSP. Fourth-year students apply for a first-year position (internship) in addition to categorical tracks for residency training. If not selected for a categorical track, it may be necessary to apply again for further residency training during the fall of your internship year, even if you plan to continue in the same program. Whether you are selected for a residency position immediately after your internship year depends on your specialty choice, level of competitiveness as an applicant, and the recommendations you receive as an intern.

All military scholarship recipients must participate in the military match. Basically, the military wants the most qualified applicant in each GME position, but several factors determine one's qualifications. Obviously, grades, board scores, research, and letters of recommendation matter, but so does the likelihood that you will remain in the service. Because of several factors, including the pay gap, the military has a difficult time retaining senior attending physicians, so they may consider the length of the student's service obligation or a history of prior service when determining who will perform an active duty residency versus being deferred to a civilian match. An unqualified applicant from USUHS will not match into a given categorical program, but instead most likely will do an internship and a General Military Officer (GMO)/Flight Surgeon tour of duty. So while a graduate of USUHS may have preference at a program because their significant obligation to the military makes them likely to stay in uniform longer, they are not guaranteed a categorical spot, just a year of active duty graduate medical education. Also, graduates of the services academies or ROTC may receive similar preferential treatment for the same reason, although they are not officially guaranteed an active duty PGY1 year.

WHAT FIRST-YEAR RESIDENCY POSITIONS ARE OFFERED IN THE MILITARY RESIDENCY MATCH?

The three military branches offer residency positions in almost all the areas offered by the civilian match, but the number of openings in any one field is limited. Family medicine, internal medicine, pediatrics, obstetrics-gynecology, surgery, psychiatry, and a transitional year are offered by all three branches.

The positions offered are based upon the needs of the military and not the desires of the applicants. While all the primary care disciplines are well represented and very obtainable for a qualified applicant, it is the subspecialties that can be limited. Specifically, neurosurgery, otolargyngology, and urology may not have any spots available during a given application year.

HOW DOES THE MILITARY MATCH FUNCTION?

Applicants list their order of preference for residency slots, and each program has its ranked list of residency applicants. Departmental representatives from each of the teaching centers meet to personally review each application. In this way, information can be exchanged about students who did active duty training at sites other than their first choice for residency. However, one student says, "as the system now works, most of the first-year internship positions are given to applicants who have completed a clerkship at the institution."

Applicants should be proactive about obtaining their residency of choice. Given that their away clerkships are paid for, the applicant should do a rotation at their desired military residency program, as this program director will be the applicant's advocate when the GME board meets.

The Navy is making an effort to give categorical spots to family medicine and psychiatry and hopes to make all residencies categorical in the future without interruption of training.

WHAT BACK-UP TASKS SHOULD YOU DO TO PREPARE FOR THE POSSIBILITY OF NOT MATCHING IN THE MILITARY?

All HPSP students may not be selected for a military residency because in some years, there are more residency applicants than positions.

All students should complete the ERAS application as soon as it is available and possibly enter the NRMP in addition to the military match program to ensure a first-year postgraduate position. If you are accepted in a military residency, you must withdraw from the NRMP with written confirmation from the Dean's office. While the NRMP fee is nonrefundable, the results of the military match are announced in early December, and you should not have to incur the costs of civilian interviews if you obtain a military residency position. Another option is to defer enrolling in the NRMP until military match day results are released and pay the $60 late registration fee in addition to the regular fee.

CAN YOU REQUEST A DEFERMENT FOR YOUR FIRST POSTGRADUATE YEAR?

The military will fill the active duty GME spots in a given specialty before granting a deferment. Some specialties have enough active duty GME positions so that all applicants will be given active duty spots. Deferments are granted if they are available for the specialty and if the applicant is determined to be competitive for the civilian match. Another factor is an applicant's expressed desire for a deferment, as no program wants a resident who does not want to be there. However, you must keep in mind that the need of the military to fill its own spots will override an applicant's personal desires.

Another class of deferment is the Civilian Sponsored spot. This is a civilian residency spot, funded by the military in which the resident is paid according to military rank. The resident will accrue an additional military obligation during this period, and these spots are very limited.

There are disadvantages to deferring as you will have less time accumulated toward promotion, pay increases, and retirement. You will not make valuable military contacts during your residency years, and you may, therefore, have less choice in your active duty assignment after you complete residency. It may also be easier to get a military fellowship after residency if your training was completed on active duty, simply because they know you and fellowship opportunities are limited.

However, while you may be 3-6 years behind in retirement, the military will still offer you the chance to stay in after the completion of your commitment, assuming a good performance.

WHAT ABOUT THE MILITARY RESERVES?

Medical students may also consider serving as a commissioned officer in the military reserves during medical school. You receive monthly drill pay for a weekend's service and the opportunity to do elective clerkships at active-duty military facilities during your third and fourth years of medical school.

Military residency positions are limited to HPSP participants and USUHS students; reservists must match in a civilian residency.

HOW DOES A CIVILIAN RESIDENT JOIN A MILITARY PROGRAM?

Military recruiters may seek civilian residents to join their programs, especially in specialty-shortage fields such as subspecialty surgery and family medicine. (Currently, there are no spots for civilians in an active duty Air Force residency). The Army offers a Financial Assistance Program, augmenting a resident's salary $1500 a month with $50,000 Education Loan Repayment. You will incur a 2-year obligation for every one year you obtain funding, paid back by participating in a variety of part-time activities your can tailor around your civilian medical practice.

The Couples Match

Scott Thomas Hadden, M.D.
Tanie Hotan, M.D.

MATCHING SUCCESSFULLY IS A COMPLICATED AND OFTEN stressful endeavor for individual applicants. This is compounded for couples, when each partner of a medical student pair hopes to match in the same geographic area. The Couples Match, a variation of the National Resident Matching Program (NRMP), was established in 1984. It allows two residency candidates graduating in the same year to pair their Rank Order Lists. Prior to 1984, a graduating couple was allowed to negotiate residency positions outside of the match or attempt to match independently through the NRMP.[1] This was an unwieldy solution, with the potential for misrepresentation on the part of both applicants and program directors. As the number of women students increased, so did the number of student couples and, likewise, the problems associated with matching. The Couples Match was introduced to address these issues.

In 1984, 812 students participated in the first Couples Match.[2] This number has increased to 808 couples or 1,616 students currently.[3] These numbers actually underestimate medical students who relocate together because some graduate in different years, and others do not use the NRMP. In 2011, 94.6 percent of couples matched successfully. This rate has remained relatively stable (Table 1).[3-4] This percentage is comparable to the match rate of individual applicants and is higher than the chance of two students matching as individuals.

HOW THE COUPLES MATCH WORKS

The Couples Match is straightforward. The Electronic Residency Application System (ERAS) allows you to designate yourself as part of a pair. This alerts programs to your situation but is not binding. The actual link between two students in the match process occurs with the submission of a Rank Order List of Paired Programs to the NRMP. This costs $15 per person in addition to the $75 registration fee. Each student can rank up to 30 different programs. After this, a fee of $30 per program is incurred. However, couples can rank as many program pairs as desired, including ones in which one student is willing to indicate "no match." You may prefer to be "unmatched" to ensure that you both will live in the same city and then try for a position later. You can create pairs of programs in any combination of specialties or geographic locations. You must both rank the same number of programs, although the "unmatched" designation is also a valid entry. More detailed instructions regarding this process can be found at www.nrmp.org.

Table 1: Recent NRMP Match Results

	2007	2008	2009	2010	2011
Applicants Who Are Coupled	1242	1476	1576	1616	1618
Matched Coupled Applicants	1106	1334	1414	1460	1478
Percent of Couples Who Matched	91.9	93.6	93.1	93.4	94.6

ADVICE FOR A SUCCESSFUL COUPLES MATCH

A successful Couples Match requires that you both know what you want from residency training, where compromises can be made, and what aspects are nonnegotiable. This includes details such as the size, setting (community versus university), and location of a program. It is crucial that you openly discuss your desires and expectations. Putting your thoughts on paper can be helpful. This reduces the likelihood of future disappointment and resentment. This is particularly important for couples entering different specialties.

When applying to programs, there are several ways to improve your chances of matching. For example, large population centers often support multiple training programs. By choosing an urban setting, you will have options to mix and match programs, giving you more combinations to put on your Rank Order List. It is also important to have a realistic understanding of your competitiveness as an applicant. You may seek advice from the Dean of Students or faculty in your specialty. In general, couples will rank more sites than their classmates. The more competitive the disciplines, the longer the rank order list is likely to be.

Another way to improve your chances of matching together is to apply early. Early in the process, programs have the most flexibility for scheduling interviews. Less competitive residencies will attempt to accommodate your timetable, whereas more competitive programs are not as flexible. Because there are more invitations than actual interview spots, you need to call and secure a time as soon as possible. We suggest that you travel together. This will allow you to compare ideas, get immediate feedback, and share expenses. Take advantage of interviewing together to show that you are a strong, stable, and well-adjusted couple.

If applying to the same residency program, you may be interviewed individually or as a pair. At the interview, inquire about the program's experience with couples. Make an effort to speak with current resident couples if there are any and even call ahead to make special arrangements. If there are no resident couples, contact recent graduates who matched as a couple. Ask about the call schedules. It would be difficult to have alternate call schedules because you would see each other mainly on post-call days. Inquire about taking vacations together. In general, the bigger the resident pool, the more accommodating the program is with vacations and call. What has worked well for some couples is to request vacation together during nonpeak times. Finally, it is enlightening to ask other residents how having a couple in their program has worked out for them.

PREGNANCY AND PARENTING

Another important couple's issue is pregnancy and parental leave. Under the NRMP guidelines, it is illegal for interviewers to initiate conversation regarding pregnancy. However, if the topic is brought up by the applicant, it can be discussed. Although there have been many programs with couples who successfully had children during their training, pregnancy is potentially disruptive for a program. The residency may be unprepared to have two residents on parental leave simultaneously, may have no formal policy for parental leave, or may have a small pool of residents to cover additional call nights. In an ideal world, every couple would be comfortable inquiring about parental leave, child care, and pregnancy issues. However, discretion should be taken because faculty and residents are not universally supportive of this issue.

SPECIAL MATCH SITUATIONS

The Couples Match was designed specifically for students entering the match at the same time and who are both applying to programs that rely on the NRMP match process. Life and love, however, are not always so conveniently arranged.

Different Medical Schools. Students graduating from different medical schools can use the NRMP. The Paired Rank Order List need not be entered at the same time or even from the same location. However, distance makes open communication more difficult.

Different Graduation Dates. Many medical student partners from the same medical school do not graduate at the same time. Unfortunately, the NRMP is unable to make provisions for these couples. However, there are several possible solutions. First, it is often feasible for the senior student to delay graduation a year in order for the couple to coordinate graduation dates. Research, fellowships, and international study are all examples of legitimate, fulfilling, and commonly employed options. If the senior cannot delay graduation, he or she can attempt to match in the same area as the medical school. If this is unsuccessful or undesirable, the junior student can take a number of rotations at or even attempt to transfer to a school close to where the partner has matched. These latter possibilities are more likely to succeed if the area is urban, with a higher density of available residency and medical school options.

Non-NRMP Programs. Several programs, for example, urology and child neurology, do not use the NRMP match but have their own independent selection process. These matches typically occur prior to the NRMP Rank Order List submission deadline. In this situation, one of you will match first. Subsequently, the other can focus rankings in the same geographic location.

PERSONAL THOUGHTS ON THE COUPLES MATCH

Matching into a residency spot is the glorious last hurdle of medical school. If you understand the logistics of the Couples Match, know what you want, apply early, and have a strong committed relationship, the Couples Match can be a successful and rewarding experience.

Things We Did Right
1. Applied early
2. Communicated openly
3. Traveled together
4. Scheduled two to three days per program
5. Spoke with resident couples

Things We Did Not Anticipate
1. Post-interview exhaustion
2. Joint interviews
3. Absence of interns during Boards Part 3 (early December)
4. Bad weather

ANOTHER COUPLE'S APPROACH

If you and your partner are applying to specialties in different matching programs, here is advice from a couple who did that. Rima Chamie, MD, applied to family medicine through the NRMP and Matt Wagner, MD, applied to urology through the American Urological Association Match.

1   Have an open discussion about the importance of matching together versus going unmatched. One woman I know decided that she would rather be with her husband and reapply the next year than live in a different city. On the other hand, some relationships didn't survive the discussions. We decided to match no matter what, and we would work out the long distance relationship if need be.

2.   Start with a separate search for locations where you are willing to live. This can be because of family, weather, medical community or whatever is important to you.

3.   Cross reference these two lists to come up with locations for application.

4.   Separate and research programs in the agreed upon locations. Make sure you have an acceptable program at which to interview in each area. For example, we had a city where one of us liked the program but the other could not find a program at which to interview. Resources and time were used on an interview that could have been skipped all together.

5.   Interviews can always be canceled. If you are offered an interview, do not wait until your partner is offered one. Schedule the interview and cancel later if you have to (always give at least 2 weeks notice).

6.   If there is a program where you are more likely to match, have your partner apply to more than one program in that location to increase chances of matching together.

7.   With the more competitive specialties, interview when you can and don't stress about being there at the same time.

8.   Tell program directors that you are trying to couples match, give them the name of your partner, and remind them later in the season. See how they respond. If they don't respect this, you may want to reconsider the program.

9.   It is also possible to work out a match together if one person is doing an "early" match such as Urology or Ophthalmology. Couples in this situation typically apply to many more programs. The advice is the same but realize that the person doing the early

match makes a list that represents what you both want. The person doing the NRMP match should finish interviewing before the early match person puts in their list so that the list can be made together. 10. Just like an exam, do not make last minute changes once you have agonized over the list. You will remember later why you didn't have it that way in the first place.

REFERENCES

1. Graettinger JS. Results of the NRMP for 1984. *J Med Educ* 1984;59:441–443.
2. Kim G. An examination of the Couples' Match. *JAMA* 1997;277(9):765.
3. Roth AE, Peranson E. The effects of the change in the NRMP Matching Algorithm. *JAMA* 1997;278(9):729–732.
4. Results and data 2011 main residency match. National Resident Matching Program, 2011 data.

What Happens if You Don't Match*

IF YOU ARE READING THIS CHAPTER, CHANCES ARE YOU ARE either a person who wants to know how to prepare for all possibilities, or you are one of the fourth-year medical students who did not match for a first-year residency position in the National Resident Matching Program (NRMP). If you are the former, I applaud your foresightedness because you will learn in this chapter about some of the preventable reasons for not matching. If you are the latter, I know that this is a stressful time and you are anxious to know what to do now.

HOW WILL I LEARN IF I DO NOT MATCH?

If you do not match, you will be informed electronically on the Monday morning of Match Week. There has been a decrease from 7.9 percent of 15,707 U.S. trained 4th-year students in 1996 to 5.9 percent of 16,559 U.S. trained 4th-year students in 2011 who participated in the NRMP but did not match. The highest fill rates in 2011 for U.S. trained 4th-year students for first-year residency positions with more than 10 positions offered by the NRMP were in vascular surgery (96.7 percent), otolaryngology (95.1 percent), dermatology (92.9 percent), plastic surgery - integrated (92.9 percent), and orthopaedic surgery (92.7 percent). The highest fill rates in 2011 for U.S. trained 4th-year

---

* I wish to thank Daniel Lowe, MD, former Associate Professor of Surgery, the Oregon Health & Sciences University School of Medicine, Frank and Ricka for assisting me in the preparation of this chapter.

students for second-year positions with more than 10 positions offered by the NRMP were radiation oncology (90.3 percent), plastic surgery (82.5 percent) and dermatology (82.3 percent).

WHAT HAPPENS IF I DO NOT MATCH?

Although actual procedures may vary from school to school, the principles involved are applicable to all unmatched students. You will find out via e-mail if you matched at 12:00 p.m. ET on the Monday of Match Week. The Dean's office may assign you to a faculty member in your preferred specialty area who will meet with you that day ,or the Dean of Student Affairs may undertake this task.

You will receive via e-mail a listing of all the openings available in the programs that offered positions through the NRMP. With the Dean of Student Affairs and/or a member of your chosen specialty's department in your school, you review your options and make a list of your preferred choices. It is helpful to have an advisor who knows about the specific programs that have openings.

Bring the following items with you in preparation for discussing your options with your faculty advisor: a copy of your ERAS application, letters of recommendation, your dean's letter, and a transcript of your grades. Also, it is important to have a road atlas (in case you need to locate an unfamiliar geographic area), and paper and pencils. A supportive spouse or partner at your side may help, especially if geographic relocation decisions have to be made.

In 2012, a new Supplemental Offer and Acceptance Program will be implemented for unmatched applicants and unfilled programs. A PowerPoint explaining the program is available at the NRMP website www.nrmp.org. Eligible applicants must use ERAS to send application to unfilled programs. They cannot use phone, fax, e-mail or other methods to send this material. Programs may start downloading applications as soon as the Supplemental Offer Application Program opens but cannot make any offers until Wednesday of Match Week. Programs will have time to review applications and conduct telephone interviews, but they cannot make any verbal offers. Residency programs will submit a second rank list of applicants to the NRMP on Wednesday morning and, beginning at noon, each unfilled program will make as many offers as there are unfilled positions for their residency to an equal number of applicants. The applicant(s) has two hours to accept or reject the offer. Applicants can receive multiple offers. If the program's offer is not accepted, the next applicant on the rank order list will receive an offer. As long as positions are available, offers will continue to be made every two hours until 6 p.m. on Wednesday, and they will start again on Thursday at 10 a.m. and continue into Friday, if necessary. Match Day ceremonies will be moved to Friday at noon ET.

HOW DID I GET IN THIS POSITION? OR HOW CAN I AVOID BEING IN THIS POSITION?

Unmatched medical students are as capable as their matched classmates. Usually errors of judgment or human factors cause these situations. Often hindsight will allow you to see how you could have prevented or at least anticipated not matching. The following cases illustrate some common causes of not matching:

John felt that he didn't need any assistance in finding a residency; after all, he had good grades and was sure that lots of emergency medicine programs would want him as a resident. He decided to aim high and ranked six of the most competitive programs. The day he was notified of his not matching, he didn't have a second choice specialty and was not aware of the options available to him.

Lisa decided to apply to surgery programs, even though her clerkship evaluation and grades were not very good. She admitted that she was not as personally aggressive as others who wished to be surgeons, and she had difficulty finding someone in the surgery department to write a letter of recommendation for her. A part-time faculty member who only worked with her twice finally agreed to write a letter on her behalf. When she did not match, only she wondered why.

Scott started early in medical school to plan for a residency match. He made sure he knew the names of the most illustrious faculty members in his medical school and went to them for his letters of recommendation, even though they had never observed his clinical skills. At each residency interview, he made sure that everyone knew that his letters were written by these famous physicians, none of whom were specialists in his field of interest. Scott was totally surprised when he did not match.

The above cases highlight the importance of getting to know physicians in the specialty to which you are applying, not just superficially, but as mentors. This, admittedly, is difficult when you may not even decide on a specialty until the end of your third year, but nothing will be lost in establishing relationships with faculty members, even if you do not choose their specialty eventually. Most faculty would rather have you choose what is right for you, rather than make a choice based on their impact as role models. Also, when you get to know them, be sure to listen to their advice—if they discourage you from entering their specialty, it is probably for a valid reason.

You may be advised not to aim too high in ranking residency programs but also to put your top choices first, even if they seem very competitive. What you may not be told is that it will be helpful to find out which programs were unfilled through the Match the prior year so you have some guidelines in ranking programs. It *is* important to only list places where you would like to live (and where a spouse or partner would like to live), but you also need to be realistic about your chances of matching. When you do your research, find out which are the most competitive residencies and be prepared to consider other programs that will offer acceptable options for the future.

A final warning: do not believe it if a program assures you that you will have a place with them. This is illegal according to Match rules, and you need to consider if you would want to spend your residency years in a program that violates these regulations.

You will be told, "If you don't match, it's not the end of the world," or some such statement. It will seem like "the end of the world" or at least the world you had anticipated. Perhaps the most helpful terminology is that used by the American Academy of Family Physicians which describes the unmatched student as a "Free Agent." With this in mind, you can accept a position that will often prove to be for you, as it has for countless others before you, a better choice than you had originally sought.

Changing Specialties During Residency and Afterwards[*]

EVERY YEAR RESIDENCY PROGRAMS RECEIVE APPLICATIONS from physicians who are in training in another specialty. Most are still in their first year; some are in later years. Some applicants are even willing to start again in the internship year. Even physicians who have practiced their specialties for several years inquire if it is possible to retrain in another specialty.

Since the demise of the "rotating internship" and the military physician draft in the mid-1970s, most medical students feel that they do not have enough information about the various specialty fields or personal insights into their own life goals. Many worry that they will find that their chosen specialty is not the "right" one. They fear that they will start their internship year and discover that their nagging doubts about their choice are increasing and that each day it will become clearer that a change must be made.

Fortunately, most of you will find that you *did* make a good choice and, in fact, realize that there isn't only "one" right choice. If you value continuity of patient care above all else, there are a number of specialties—e.g., family medicine, general pediatrics, general internal medicine, psychiatry—in which you have the opportunity to establish long-term relationships with patients. If research is what excites you,

---

[*] Modification of an article originally published in *Consultant* 1990;30(2):14–25. Used with permission.

there are questions to answer in every specialty. If you are energized in the operating room, a number of fields will allow you to spend your professional time in that setting.

Even the most content physician will have days, however, when specialty choice is questioned. This happens commonly during the stressful residency years. A study[1] showed that "self-doubt about choice of specialty" was reported by 28.8 percent of the 234 first-year resident respondents. While the percentage expressing "self-doubt" decreased to 19 percent in the second year and 12 percent in the third, it increased to 17.6 percent in the fourth year and remained at this high level (16.7 percent) even into the sixth year of postgraduate training.

Ideally, the specialty you choose will be the one you truly prefer. Matteson and Smith[2] have postulated that there is a difference between specialty preference and choice. In their study of 350 medical students, they ascertained that 25 percent of their sample reported a specialty choice other than their preferred one. Reasons given for choosing a specialty that was not "preferred" involved concerns about lifestyle (the preferred specialty would demand too much) and finances (the preferred specialty would not be lucrative enough to repay educational loans quickly). Sex differences may also be a factor in choice as women perceive certain specialties, such as surgery, as being "male strongholds" and the necessary dedication to succeed in such a field may seem to be overwhelming. If you do not choose your "preferred" specialty for reasons such as the need to mesh dual careers, an image of yourself that proves to be unrealistic, advice—perhaps misguided— that you are not academically qualified to match in a desired specialty, someday you may say, "This is not what I want to do with my life."

WHO CHANGES SPECIALTIES?

The Association of American Medical Colleges (AAMC) has initiated longitudinal studies of specialty switching during residency years. A study[3] that followed the 1983 medical school class found that by the end of the third year of residency, 13 percent had changed from their original specialty field. An earlier study[4] found that by the fifth postgraduate year, 10 percent of the 106 graduates surveyed had switched specialties. Eleven percent of U.S. residents in a first-year residency position in 1997 had already received prior residency training and were changing specialties.[5] These figures indicate that the number of residents changing specialties has remained relatively stable. It is also evident that changing specialties is not a new phenomenon.

Are there any identifiable personality traits shared by the physicians changing specialties? The Myers-Briggs Type Indicator is the basis of a longitudinal study of 5355 physicians tested in the early 1950s and then evaluated in 1963 and 1973 to specifically examine changes in specialties.[6] Results indicate that physicians tended to change to a "more typical specialty" (one more reflective of their personality type). For example, an action-oriented person who valued independence was more likely to change to emergency medicine than to stay in internal medicine. In addition, those who strongly needed a sense of personal fulfillment in their work were more likely to change specialties than those who desired a stable and secure future.

IS THERE A "BEST TIME" TO CHANGE?

Yes, as soon as possible, for the well-being of both the individual and the residency program. In one program,[7] 75 percent of the first-year residents left, although not all to switch specialties. From a program director's point of view, this is most distressing, "If I cannot fill a vacancy, service commitments cannot be fully met and the morale of remaining residents is diminished."

A vacancy in the third year can be particularly difficult for family medicine residencies, where a resident must spend the final two years of training in the same program to be eligible for board certification. This precludes the possibility of filling a third-year vacancy.

HOW DOES A RESIDENT CHANGE TO ANOTHER SPECIALTY?

Before making a specialty change, you should ask yourself some specific questions to clarify your personal and professional goals:

Why did I choose medicine as a career?

What did I imagine myself doing in medicine when I entered medical school?

What messages (spoken and unspoken) about my specialty choice do I receive from my family?

What do I want from my career, and how will I know when I achieve it?

How do I define success?

Can I contribute more to the specialty I am considering than to the one I originally chose?

If you decide to change specialties during your first year of residency, you will spend time during the early Spring calling programs and applying to those that know they will have vacancies and are of interest to you. You may need to take vacation time in order to schedule interviews. The hardest part will involve your personal relationships: your family, especially if it involves geographic relocation; your class of interns, who usually become a close group even in a short period of time; and your program director and faculty physician attendings, who chose you to join them in the residency.

Changing in later years of residency is increasingly problematic. In addition to your own feelings of having invested time training and wondering if it will all be "wasted," there are some very real economic constraints. Medicare payments to hospitals for educational costs were significantly reduced in 1989–1990. A formula is used to calculate the per-resident reimbursement of educational costs to hospitals. Full payments are made only for residents whose ". . . total years of training are no more than required to meet initial specialty board qualifications plus one year with a maximum of five years." The hospital receives less reimbursement for residents whose total training is beyond those limits. The initial residency period is established at entry to your first residency program. So if you first match in surgery, your initial residency period is set at 5 years; you can change to a residency requiring 3 or 4 years for board certification, and the hospital will not lose any Medicare funding.[8] At least one hospital[9] has made it a policy to require any program that appoints residents for whom full Medicare payment will not be received to reimburse the hospital for the difference in costs. This effectively means that in this hospital, a three-year program, such as family practice or internal medicine, would have to pay a portion of the salary of any resident who has previously completed two years or more of another specialty's residency. If you are currently in your second or third year of residency, it is probable that a residency program in this hospital would be reluctant to consider your application.

WHY DO PHYSICIANS MAKE SPECIALTY CHANGES?

Included in some studies' statistics are physicians who planned to change specialties after the first year of residency, using the first year of internal medicine or surgery to prepare for training in radiology or a surgical subspecialty. To a decreasing degree, some may plan to obtain licensure after the required year of internship and enter general or emergency room practice.

During the stressful first year of residency, escape from a "bad situation" may be the motivating factor in a specialty change. Views of the specialty may be unrealistically negative. Or the residency program may be undergoing changes that impact your perception of the specialty. It is important to get as full a picture of what is making you feel unhappy with your specialty choice as possible. Escaping to another specialty training program may not be the answer. Ideally, you should come to the conclusion that your desire to change is coming from personal self-assessment and a desire to do something else in medicine rather than from a need to flee a "bad situation."

Financial indebtedness may enter into your specialty choice decision. Some physicians switch to shorter residencies so they can enter the marketplace sooner. Trying to guess which specialties will be favored by future reimbursement plans clouds the more important issue: you will have to practice your chosen specialty long after all your school debts are paid.

In later years of residency and practice, a specialty change is even more difficult as more years have been invested in the original choice and your identity as a member of a particular branch of medicine has been even more firmly established in everyone's mind. Your leaving may be interpreted by colleagues as rejection; at the very least, it will make them uncomfortable. However, your personal discomfort may be so overwhelming that a change is mandatory for your continued well-being.

AN ALTERNATIVE TO CHANGING SPECIALTIES

If you have a strong quest for "competence" in areas of medicine that are increasingly complex and technical, you might initially seek training in multiple specialties. Some institutions are offering programs that provide simultaneous training in two fields, such as combined residencies in pediatrics and internal medicine; emergency medicine and internal medicine; and pediatrics, psychiatry, and child psychiatry.

If you have already committed to a specialty, you should consider if you can find a "niche" within your chosen specialty that will be fulfilling. The "emerging specialty areas" discussed in Part 3 of the book are examples of career options in which physicians are building on their past training to find new challenges. Primary care physicians are narrowing their practice focus, perhaps to an age group such as adolescents or a medical problem, such as chronic pain; all types of specialists are entering administrative medicine. Or, you might find that what needs to be changed is your practice setting rather than your specialty; joining a group practice or accepting a salaried position may rejuvenate your professional life. A short-term break (called a sabbatical in academics) may be all that is needed—perhaps, time spent as a medical missionary to a developing country or a locum tenens (temporary substitute for an absent practicing physician) in this country.

Whatever your decision, it is important to include family members in your assessment and planning. Change of any kind will be easier if they understand why it is necessary and are involved in the process. Only then will you achieve the fulfillment and success you seek in your medical career.

REFERENCES

1. Taylor AD, Sinclair AS, Wall EM. Sources of stress in post-graduate medical training. *J Med Educ* 1987;62:425–428.
2. Matteson MT, Smith SV. Selection of medical specialties: Preference versus choices. *J Med Educ* 1977;52:548–554.
3. Dial TH, Lindley DW. Predictive validity of specialty choice data from AAMC graduation questionnaire. *J Med Educ* 1987;62:955–958.
4. Wasserman E, Yufit RI, Pollock GH. Medical specialty choice and personality. *Arch Gen Psychiat* 1969;21:529–535.
5. Dunn MR, Miller RS, Richter TH. Graduate medical education 1997–1998. *JAMA* 1998;280(9):809–818.
6. McCaulley MH. The Myers Longitudinal Medical Study. Monograph II, Contract No. 231-76-0051, Health Resources Administration, DHEW, Gainesville, Florida: Center for Applications of Psychological Type, 1977.
7. Davidson RC, Brown TC, Ramirez-Rude A. A review of resident drop-outs from a family practice residency network. *Fam Med* 1981;13(4):10–13.
8. Beall D. Graduate medical education financing and its effect on residency program choice change, Part 1. *JAMA* 1997;277(8):612.
9. Clark WM. Internal memorandum. Portland, Oregon: Oregon Health Sciences University School of Medicine, November 18, 1988.

APPENDIX

Questionnaire

1. When did you choose your medical specialty? (Check one) Did a person or event influence you?

    _____ Before entering medical school

    _____ During medical school

    _____ During internship year

    _____ During residency

    _____ Other (please specify)

2. Specifically what appealed to you about your chosen specialty?
3. What do you enjoy *most* about your work?
4. What do you enjoy *least* about your work?
5. Describe a "typical" day: how many hours of work, types of activities, types of problems seen most often, patient population?
6. Describe additional professional duties: on-call schedule, continuing education, and/or hospital meetings.
7. What abilities or talents are important in your specialty?
8. What personality traits best characterize the practitioners of your specialty?
9. What advice would you give a medical student interested in your specialty?
10. What are the future challenges to your specialty?
11. What other specialty fields did you think of entering and why didn't you?

12. What field would you *not* want to practice and why?

13. Choose four of the following job values that are most important to you:

_____ Creativity   _____ Independence
_____ Good income   _____ Decision making
_____ Variety   _____ Prestige
_____ Security   _____ Achievement
_____ Working with people   _____ Sufficient time off
_____ Working with my hands   _____ Feedback from others
_____ Working with my mind   _____ Taking care of people

14. Check one in each of the following statements:

I prefer   ___ a known routine   ___ the unexpected
People   ___ energize me   ___ exhaust me
I am more   ___ serious and determined
                       ___ easy going

Immediate gratification and feedback is
                       ___ very important   ___ not very important

I am more often
                       ___ cool-headed   ___ warm-hearted

I am more interested in
                       ___ what is actual   ___ what is possible

With patients I prefer
                       ___ long-term   ___ short-term relationships

I tend to   ___ be good at   ___ dislike precise work

I am a   ___ thoughtful realist
                      ___ thoughtful innovator
                      ___ action-oriented realist
                      ___ action-oriented innovator

First-Year Postgraduate Positions Offered Through the National Resident Matching Program (NRMP)

Anesthesiology
Dermatology
Emergency Medicine
Family Medicine
General Surgery
Internal Medicine
Medical Genetics
Neurological Surgery
Neurology
Obstetrics-Gynecology
Ophthalmology
Orthopaedic Surgery
Otolaryngology
Pathology
Pediatrics
Physical Medicine and Rehabilitation
Plastic Surgery
Preventive Medicine
Psychiatry
Radiation Oncology
Radiology-Diagnostic
Transitional
Urology

Summary Profile Scores

You can complete the questionnaires and obtain your scores for all specialties online at www.sdn.net. Alternatively, after reading each chapter and completing its questionnaire, enter your summary scores here:

Allergy and Immunology____

Anesthesiology ____

Colon and Rectal Surgery ____

Dermatology ____

Emergency Medicine ____

Family Medicine____

General Internal Medicine ____

Cardiology ____

Endocrinology and Metabolism ____

Gastroenterology ____

Hematology ____

Infectious Diseases ____

Medical Oncology ____

Nephrology ____

Pulmonary Disease ____

Rheumatology ____

Medical Genetics ____

Neurological Surgery ____

Neurology ____
Nuclear Medicine ____
Obstetrics-Gynecology ____
Ophthalmology ____
Orthopaedic Surgery ____
Otolaryngology ____
Pathology ____
Pediatrics ____
Physical Medicine and Rehabilitation ____
Plastic Surgery ____
Aerospace Medicine ____
Occupational Medicine ____
Public Health and General Preventive Medicine ____
Psychiatry ____
Radiation Oncology ____
Radiology, Diagnostic ____
Surgery ____
Thoracic Surgery ____
Urology ____

Selected Web Sites

American Medical Association (AMA)	http://www.ama-assn.org
American Medical Student Association (AMSA)	http://www.amsa.org
Association of American Medical Colleges (AAMC)	http://www.aamc.org
Association of Hospital Medical Education (list of transitional residency programs)	http://www.ahme.med.edu
Career MD (residency and fellowship database)	http://www.careermd.com
Electronic Residency Application Service (ERAS)	http://www.aamc.org
Fellowship and Residency Electronic Interactive Database Access (FREIDA)	http://www.ama-assn.org/freida
Internship and Residency Information Site	http://www.I-r-I-s.com
National Resident Matching Program (NRMP)	http://aamc.org/nrmp
Official USMLE Information	http://www.usmle.org
Osteopathic Rotations and Residency Resource	http://www.studentdo.com
ResidencySite.com	http://www.residencysite.com
Student Doctor Network	http://www.sdn.net
Scutwork.com	http://www.scutwork.com

Index

X